Business Essentials for Nurse Practitioners

Essential Knowledge for Building Your Practice

Dr. Kevin Lee Letz

Published by PreviCare, Inc. Publishing

For information, please contact:
PreviCare, Inc.
2602 Barry Knoll Way
Suite 300
Fort Wayne, In. 46845

This book has been published to provide accurate and
authoritative information in regard to the subject matter
covered. It is sold with the understanding that the
publisher and author are not engaged in rendering legal,
accounting, or other professional advice. If legal, financial
or other expert assistance is required, the services of a
competent professional should be sought.

ISBN: 0-9714762-8-4

Printed in the United States of America

Dedication

To Michelle and all her extremely hard work.

Business Essentials for Nurse Practitioners

4

Table of Contents

Business Essentials for Nurse Practitioners
6

Preface

The healthcare field is undergoing drastic changes, and whether we like it or not, business professionals are now driving how we as providers deliver health care services. We all know how important it is to maintain clinical skills and knowledge. I believe it is also now important to learn the business of being a clinician. I wrote this book because now is a time that every health care professional including nurse practitioners needs to have business savvy in addition to knowledge regarding patient care. I did not write this book to give you legal guidance. I am not a lawyer or an expert in business. I consider myself an expert in health and wellness just like you and most practitioners. I have found it essential to know aspects of business practice to succeed and practice effectively. I am merely sharing some of my business knowledge with you so that you too can practice effectively and succeed in your own career. Nurse practitioners have proven that they provide quality care and are cost effective. I think what we have lacked as a profession is the business savvy to sell ourselves and effectively communicate our worth. In summation, clinicians who do not understand business principles as they relate to medical practice are in danger of becoming ineffective healers. This book provides the essential business knowledge NP's must have to respond to emerging challenges in a proactive way, rather than with fear and disappointment.

Business Essentials for Nurse Practitioners
8

Chapter 1

The Role of the NP in the Current Health Care Environment

"Great minds discuss ideas; average minds discuss events, small minds discuss people." *Author unknown*

Many Americans contend that the U.S. health care system is in serious disarray. The U.S. spends far more per capita on health care than nearly all other industrialized nations but at the same time is looked upon as the best among the citizens of these same countries. Improving the current health care system will take a "mental set" that integrates clinical and financial information. In addition to the high cost of care provided in the U.S. other problems have been identified including poor accessibility to those with less financial means and a focus on illness and disease management rather than prevention and wellness services. The shortage of primary care physicians in the 1960's brought about the role of the nurse practitioner and physician assistant to provide care to those having difficulty obtaining primary care services. Since that time these clinicians have provided high quality services in a cost effective manner. Obviously, the expansion of the NP and PA professions can *assist* in correcting the majority of health care problems in the U.S. with the help of physicians and legislators.

Any type of reformed health care system will be forced to function with both fewer physicians and nurses than the current system unless universities see a dramatic upswing in enrollment. Nurse practitioners will no doubt be an important part of the new health care system no matter how it is formulated, however, in what facet will have to be determined.

Healthcare consumers are much different than they were just 5 to 10 years ago. Consumers are now taking more control of their care and are demanding freedom of choice in providers even if they are given a list to choose from. Health care consumers and the media are placing more emphasis on health promotion and illness prevention. However, the majority of consumers including the media do not know that this is the forte of the nurse practitioner. Nurse practitioners are trained not only to manage the common presenting illnesses and disease processes encountered in primary care but also in the arts of providing patient education and counseling. Nurse practitioners also have the tremendous ability to build relationships with their patients increasing both patient satisfaction and quality of care.

The baby boomers are coming of age and at the same time the United States is beginning to experience the beginning of a physician shortage. Many experts believe there will be a shortage of over 200,000 physicians by the year 2020. Additionally, 2 of 3 physicians today are specialists. The shortage of primary care physicians may open up barriers/restrictions to practice for nurse practitioners. At the same time there exists a nursing shortage of nearly 200,000 that is expected to climb to 400,000 by the year 2020. The Bureau of Health Professions announced in February of 2001 that there are over 88,000 nurse practitioners in the United States. NP's should reach numbers as high as 200,000 by 2020.

The majority of nurse practitioners today practice in the traditional primary care specialties including family practice, pediatrics and ob-gyn practices. The increased complexity of patients and increasing number of specialty-trained physicians also creates the need for nurse practitioners in a variety of direct care roles in further specialized arenas. The market for NP's in acute care will increase as economists continue to keep a close eye on health care costs and funding of graduate medical education programs dries up.

Competition or Collaboration?

Both. Competition is important in any business. If we really want to improve access to care and cut spending then we should ensure fair competition in the medical marketplace. Laws should guarantee a patient's right to choose among all qualified health professionals, not just HMO participating physicians. Congress and the White House should break up the medical monopoly that protects doctors from competition (which exists in nearly all other types of business) by other health professionals who are just as qualified to meet the majority of our health care needs. Physicians should not have a monopoly on health care because they certainly do not have a monopoly on the knowledge of providing health care. Nurse practitioners can more than adequately provide the majority of duties involved in primary care and can be trained at 1/5th the cost.

The role of the physician will continue to grow and they will never find themselves without work. Physicians will continually be needed to care for the truly ill patients who require more invasive testing and treatment modalities. Nurse practitioners will never threaten this role. Nurse practitioners will continue to fulfill the role of health maintenance, treatment of acute uncomplicated illness and the maintenance of chronic disease. This role is an area physicians are often choosing not to do. Complicated cases and conditions can easily be referred to a primary care physician or specialist in a similar way primary care physicians refer to specialists.

Critical Initiatives for NP's

There are three critical initiatives NP's must take while the health care system continues to undergo change:

    A. Continue to do what we do best.

Providing high quality, cost conscious, patient centered care with a high level of patient satisfaction is what NP's do best and must continue to do above all else.

    B. Market our role.

Expanding the knowledge of our existence to the public and other health care professionals is something we have not done well and thus must improve. Remember that in this country the consumer will eventually have the largest say in the way the health care system evolves. Discussing our role with everyone we come into contact with will ultimately advance our profession the greatest.

    C. Foster true collaboration

Fostering true collaboration with our physician counterparts may be difficult since physicians have historically been practicing with limited competition. Educate physicians about how they can work with NP's to provide higher quality care collaboratively.

Business Essentials for Nurse Practitioners
14

Chapter 2

Certification and Licensure

"NP education is not completed at graduation"

What is the difference?

Regulation of a medical professional can be
accomplished either through licensure of certification.
Licensure is publicly controlled by the state or
governing authority which sets minimum standards for
the profession in order for a person to practice under
such title. The Constitution has delegated the states to
oversee the licensure process and maintenance.
Certification can be considered more of an option for
the individual practitioner in that it is not necessary for
practice but can often be required for certain rights of
practice such as prescriptive authority or government
and third party payment. Certification always requires
testing to establish certain high level knowledge in a
particular field of study. Certification is usually
monitored by nongovernmental agencies that are often a
specialty organization in the field of the certification.
Becoming certified is often a statement that whoever is
certified in a specialty area is an expert in that
particular field of study. The American Nurses
Credentialing Center (ANCC) defines certification as the
"process in which an organization, based on
predetermined standards, validates an RN's
qualifications, knowledge, and practice in a functional
or clinical area of nursing" (1).

Becoming Certified

Several organizations offer certification for advanced
practice nurses (Table 2-1). Currently, states and
organizations that require certification do not
distinguish which organizations are preferred.

Table 2-1

Organizations Offering NP Certification

Organization Cost	Certification
AANP www.aanp.org Cost: Member $185, Nonmember $270	Family NP, Adult NP
ANCC www.nursingworld.org/ancc Cost: Member $230, Discount rate $300, Nonmember $370	Family NP, Adult NP, Gerontological NP, Pediatric NP, School NP, Acute Care NP (in conjunction with American Association of Critical Care Nurses Certification Corp.)
National Certification Corporation for the Obstetrical, Gynecologic, and Neonatal NP Nursing Specialties www.nccnet.org Cost: $250	Neonatal NP Women's Health NP
National Certification Board of Pediatric NP's www.pnpcert.org Cost: $375	Pediatric NP

The certifying organizations are moving toward the requirement of a master's degree or higher in nursing. Each of the organizations has their own requirements in order to sit for their exams and can be obtained by contacting the organizations. The ANCC and AANP offer computerized testing which shortens the testing time and also allows for easier access to testing sites. Many people still prefer the pencil and paper exams however

and these are available from some of the certifying
bodies.

Preparing for Certification

You know better than anyone else your best method of
preparation for an exam. The certification exams are no
different. Several organizations are set up to assist you
in your studies with study books, tapes, and seminars.

Staying Certified

American Nurses Credentialing Center (ANCC)

The ANCC requires NP's to re-certify every 5 years. The
ANCC requires the NP to practice a minimum of 1,500
hours during the certification period. Nursing faculty
may fulfill part of this requirement through didactic and
clinical teaching. A minimum of 75 contact hours of
continuing education is necessary for re-certification.
Alternatively five academic semester hours or six
academic quarter hours may be used. The ANCC also
requires that 51% of your continuing education must be
directly related to the specialty area of certification and
academic courses must be applicable to the area of
certification as well. Beginning January 1st of 2003, at
least 50% of continuing education credits must be
obtained through ANCC approved providers. Re-
certification will require one of the following categories:
Category 1: 25 contact hours, Category 2: 2 semester
hours or 3 quarter hours, Category 3: 10 different
presentations, Category 4: 1 published book chapter or
article, 1 research project, 1 other educational media
project, or a doctoral dissertation or master's thesis in
the specialty are of certification, Category 5: 150 hours
of clinical preceptorship of graduate level advanced
practice students. You may also choose to re-certify by
re-examination following the same requirements as

someone taking their initial examination. There is not a special re-certification examination.

American Academy of Nurse Practitioners (AANP)

The AANP requires NP's to re-certify every 5 years. Re-certification requires a minimum of 1,000 practice hours during the certification period along with 75 earned contact hours of continuing education relevant to the area of specialization. The NP seeking re-certification through re-examination must take the same examination as the first-time examinee and meet the same eligibility standards.

The certifying agencies should send you notice that your certification period is about to end but do not rely on this.

Hospital Privileges

Professional staff privileges often include the right to admit, treat, or consult on the clinical treatment of patients within the hospital setting. Less than 15% of nurse practitioners report having clinical staff privileges allowing them to admit and care for their own patients. While laws are usually quite lenient with regard to privileges for nurse practitioners and their practice in the hospital environment, hospitals often impose restrictions on privileges for non-physician providers. The Joint Commission on Accreditation of Healthcare Organizations (JCAHO) of which the majority of hospitals participate in does not require hospitals to grant privileges to nurse practitioner but does not disallow it. State laws vary but generally will allow privileges for nurse practitioners at some level. In most circumstances then it is up to the hospital whether they allow the granting of privileges to nurse practitioners.

Obtaining hospital privileges is a process known as credentialing. The credentialing process usually begins by filling out an application for staff privileges and then later review by a medical staff board often consisting of physicians. Applications are similar to what is seen when applying for a Medicare number but often requires a few references and more specifics with regard to previous employment. Generally speaking, there are two types of clinical privileges. Full privileges grant the practitioner to admit, write orders, discharge etc. without supervision or co-signature of a physician. Full privileges are rarely granted to nurse practitioners. Associate or extender privileges allow varying degrees of privileges but usually require direct oversight by a sponsoring physician. This form of privileges is what is most frequently given to the traditional "rounding nurse" or "physician extender". Certainly, the formation of a separate type of privilege for nurse practitioners would not be out of the question. Ideally, allowing more autonomy than associate privileges yet some degree of oversight with a hospitalist or collaborating physician similar to what occurs in the outpatient setting.

Having hospital privileges has its pros and cons that should be reviewed before deciding whether to take on this additional role. A few benefits of hospital privileges include heightening the awareness of nurse practitioners, maintaining continuity of care for your patients, and a chance to shift some responsibility off your collaborating physician and thus further increase your value to the practice. The drawbacks to having hospital privileges include the additional work, responsibility and risk that come along with such privileges. Rarely, are nurse practitioners remunerated for the additional work involved with hospital care. Your decision on whether to obtain privileges should be based on the pros and cons above and your comfort level with hospital based care.

Professional Memberships

Belonging to specialty organization has tremendous benefits including continuing education opportunities, networking, some degree of prestige, and a resource for further information. For most, it is not financially possible to join every nurse practitioner organization that exists, so some thought must go into your decision of which organizations to join.

National Nurse Practitioner Organizations

American Academy of Nurse Practitioners
Capitol Station, LBJ Building
P.O. Box. 12846
Austin, TX 78711
(512) 442-4626
www.aanp.org

American College of Nurse Practitioners
1111 19th Street, NW, Suite 404
Washington, D.C. 20036
(202) 659-2190
www.nurse.org/acnp

National Association of Pediatric Nurse Practitioners
1101 Kings Hwy. North, Suite 206
Cherry Hill NJ 08034-1012
(609) 667-1773
www.napnpa.org

Association of Women's Health, Obstetric, & Neonatal
Nurses
2000 L Street, Suite 740
Washington, D.C. 20036
(800) 673-8449
www.awhonn.org

National Alliance of Nurse Practitioners
325 Pennsylvania Avenue, SE
Washington, D.C. 20003
(202) 675-6350

National Association of Nurse Practitioners in Women's
Health
503 Capitol Court, NE, Suite 300
Washington, D.C.   20002
(202) 543-9693
www.npwh.org

National Conference of Gerontological Nurse
Practitioners
P.O. Box 232230
Centreville, VA 2012-2230
(703) 802-0088
www.ncgnp.org

National Organization of Nurse Practitioner Faculties
1522 K Street NW, Suite 702
Washington, D.C. 20005
(202) 289-8044
www.nonpf.com

American College of Nurse Midwives
818 Connecticut Ave. NW, Suite 900

Washington DC 20036
(202) 728-9897
www.midwife.org

Association of Advanced Practice Psychiatric Nurses
5550 33rd Ave. NE Seattle, WA 98105
(206) 524-4090
www.aappn.org

Uniformed Nurse Practitioner Association
1153 Bergen Pkwy., Suite M-181
Evergreen, CO 80439
(800) 759-2881
www.unpa.org

State Nurse Practitioner Organizations

Alaska Nurse Practitioner Association
237 E. Third Ave. Suite 3
Anchorage, AK 99501
(907) 222-6847 www.alaskanp.org

Arizona Nurse Practitioner Council-Pheonix
1850 E. Southern Ave., Suite 1
Tempe, AZ 85282
(480) 831-0404

Southern Arizona Nurse Practitioners
10981 N Black Canyon Ct.
Oro Valley AZ 85737
(520) 544-9606
www.nurse.org/az/sanp

Arkansas Department of Health Nurse Practitioners Group
200 S. University, Suite 310
Little Rock, AR 72204
(501) 663-6080

Arkansas Nurses Association and Council of Advanced Practice Nursing
804 N. University
Little Rock, AR 72205
(501) 664-5953
www.arna.org

California Coalition of Nurse Practitioners
2300 Bethards Dr., Suite K
Santa Rosa, CA 95405
(707) 575-8090
www.ccnp.org

Connecticut Nurse Practitioner Group, Inc.
2842 Main St., #323
Glastonbury, CT 06033
www.nurse.org/ct/cnpgi

Advanced Practice Nurse Council of the Delaware Nurses Association
2644 Capitol Tail
Neward, DE 29722
(302) 368-2333
www.deapn.org

Nurse Practitioner Association of DC
PO Box 9718
Washington, DC 20016-9718
(202) 686-5514
www.npadc.org

Florida Nurses Association
PO Box 536985
Orlando, FL 32853-6985
(407) 896-3261
www.floridanurse.org

Georgia Nurse Practitioner Council
3032 Briarcliff Rd.
Atlanta, GA 30329
(404) 325-5536

Nurse Practitioner Council of Coastal GA
PO Box 14046
Savannah, GA 31416
(912) 351-7800

Nurse Practitioner Conference Group of Idaho
(208) 853-8426

Illinois Nurses Association, Council of Advanced Practice Nurses
4431 S. Raymond Ave.
Brookfield, IL 60513
(312) 692-3032
www.illinoisadvancednurses.org

Coalition of Advanced Practice Nurses of Indiana
233 McCrea St.
Indianapolis, IN 46225
www.capni.org

Iowa Association of Nurse Practitioners
College of Nursing, University of Iowa
Iowa City, IA 52242
(319) 335-9990
www.iowaanp.org

Iowa Nurse Practitioner Society
53 Norwood Circle
Iowa City, IA 52245-5024
(319) 338-8189
www.iowanpsociety.com

Kansas Alliance of Advanced NP's
8100 E. 22nd Street Bldg.
1500-B Wichita, KS 67226-2315
(316) 682-5900

Kentucky Coalition of Nurse Practitioners and Nurse Midwives
171 Louisiana Ave
Lexington, KY 40502
(859) 266-5542
www.kcnpnm.org

Louisiana Association of NP's
1501 Bethia Street
Franklin, LA 70538
(337) 828-7526
www.lanp.org

Maine Nurse Practitioner Association
11 Columbia Street
Augusta, ME 04330
(207) 621-0313

Nurse Practitioner Association of Maryland
Annapolis, MD 21404-0701
(888) 405-NPAM
www.nurse.org/md/npam

Massachusetts Coalition of NP's
PO Box 1153
Littleton, MA 01460

(781) 575-1565
www.mcnpweb.org

Mississippi Nurses Association NP Special Interest Group
31 Woodgreen Place
Madison, MS 39110
(601) 898-0670
www.msnnurses.org

Arkansas-Missouri Association of NP's
PO Box 824
Kenneth, MO 63857-0824
(573) 888-0038

Nevada Nurses' Association Nurse Practitioner Group
4753 Lake Place
Las Vegas, NV 89117

New Hampshire NP Association
PO Box 833
Concord, NH 03302-0833
(603) 648-2233
www.npweb.org

Forum for Nurses in Advanced Practice, New Jersey
State Nurses Association 1479 Pennington Road
Trenton, NJ 08618 (609) 883-5335
www.nurse.org/nj/njsna

New Mexico Nurse Practitioner Council
7317 Mayflower Drive, NE
Albuquerque, NM 87109   (505)
821-3461

New York State Coalition of Nurse Practitioners, Inc.
113 Great Oaks Blvd.
Albany, NY 12203
(518) 456-8935

North Carolina Nurses Association Council of NP's
PO Box 12025
Raleigh, NC 27605-2025
(919) 821-4250
www.ncnurses.org

Oklahoma Nurse Practitioners
404 North Main Street
Seminole, OK 74868
(405) 382-2627
www.oknp.org

Nurse Practitioners of Oregon
18768 SW Boones, Ferry Road
Tualatin, OR 97062
www.npo.oregonrn.org

Pennsylvania Coalition of Nurse Practitioners
893 Stone Jug Road
Biglerville, PA 17307

Advanced Practice Registered Nurse Council of the South Carolina Nurses Association
1821 Gadsden Columbia, SC 29201
(803) 779-3870
www.scnurses.org

Nurse Practitioner Association of South Dakota
2715 Jackson Blvd.
Rapid City, SD 57401
(605) 341-3554
www.usd.edu/npasd

Tennessee Nurses Association Council of Advanced Practice Nurses
545 Mainstream Drive, Suite 405
Nashville, TN 37228-1296

(615) 254-03510
www.tnaonline.org

Texas Nurse Practitioners
305 Spring Creek Village, PMB 618
Dallas, TX 75248
(972) 404-3035
www.texasnp.org

Vermont NP Associates Inc.
PO Box 64773
Burlington, VT 05401

Virginia Council of Nurse Practitioners
3108 N Parham Road, Suite 200B
Richmond, VA 23294 (804) 346-4840
www.virginianurses.com

ARNP's United of Washington State
10024 SE 240th Street, Suite 102
Kent WA 98031
(253) 480-1035
www.nurse.org/wa/au

Metro Milwaukee Nurse Practitioners
PO Box 13674
Wauwatosa, WI 53213-0674
(414) 297-9416

Wisconsin Nurse Practitioners in Women's Health
2025 E. Greenwich #201
Milwaukee, WI 53211
(414) 332-8590

Business Essentials for Nurse Practitioners
30

Chapter 3

Prescriptive and Legal Authority for Nurse Practitioners

Always ask yourself; "Is there any reason why the patient shouldn't receive this drug?"

Prescriptive Authority for Nurse Practitioners

Prescriptive authority for nurse practitioners has been a key factor in the credibility and expansion of the nurse practitioner role. Without prescriptive authority it would be difficult for nurse practitioners to become primary care providers or to function in any independent fashion. The expansion of prescriptive authority has and will likely continue to be met with resistance. While physicians focus their attention on the expansion of nursing roles other professions are looking for in roads including pharmacists and psychologists.

There are no states that do not address prescriptive authority for nurse practitioners. Following is a summary of prescriptive authority among all states. Individual state regulation may change and it is important to check with your state board of nursing for current authority. Contact your state board of nursing for requirements in obtaining prescriptive authority. The Drug Enforcement Agency (DEA) recently placed application forms online for NP's to apply for DEA numbers for those who live in states where this is granted (www.deadversion.usdoj.gov).

States were NP's may prescribe with physician involvement or delegation of prescriptive writing by a physician. NP's may not prescribe controlled substances in theses states.

Alabama, Florida, Kentucky, Missouri, Nevada, Texas.

States were NP's may prescribe with physician involvement or delegation of prescription writing by a physician. NP's may prescribe controlled substances in these states.

Alabama, California, Colorado, Connecticut, Delaware, Hawaii, Idaho, Illinois, Indiana, Kansas, Maryland, Massachusetts, Michigan, Minnesota, North Carolina, North Dakota, New Jersey, New York, Ohio, Oklahoma, Pennsylvania, Rhode Island, South Carolina, South Dakota, Tennessee, Virginia, Vermont, West Virginia, Iowa, Utah, Wyoming, Mississippi, Louisiana.

States were NP's may prescribe independently of a physician. Controlled Substances may be prescribed as well.

Alaska, Arizona, Maine, Montana, New Hampshire, New Mexico, Oregon, Washington, Wisconsin, District of Columbia.

In Georgia, NP's can call in prescriptions but may not write them yet under their name.

Scope of Practice For Nurse Practitioner's.

States where the board of nursing has sole authority in scope of practice with no need for physician collaboration or oversight.

Alaska, Arkansas, Arizona, Colorado, District of Columbia, Hawaii, Iowa, Kansas, Kentucky, Maine, Michigan, Montana, North Dakota, New Hampshire, New Jersey, New Mexico, Oklahoma, Oregon, Rhode Island, Texas, Utah, Washington, West Virginia, Wyoming.

States where the board of nursing has sole authority in scope of practice, but the scope of practice requires physician collaboration.

Connecticut, Delaware, Illinois, Indiana, Ohio, Maryland, Minnesota, Missouri, Nebraska, Nevada, New York, Vermont, Wisconsin.

States where the board of nursing has sole authority in scope of practice, but the scope of practice requires physician supervision.

California, Florida, Georgia, Idaho, Louisiana, Massachusetts, South Carolina.

States where the scope of practice is authorized by both the board of nursing and board of medicine.

Alabama, Mississippi, North Carolina, Pennsylvania, South Dakota, Virginia.

**States where NP's function under a broad
nurse practice act.**

Tennessee.

Business Essentials for Nurse Practitioners
36

Chapter 4

Searching, Landing, and Starting a New Position

"Never talk negatively about present or previous employers during an interview"

Employment Options for NP's

Clinicians entering practice today are confronted with a more complicated business environment than years past. The increase in business complexity results from the rapid restructuring of health care delivery that may open up new and different opportunities to clinicians. Given the multitude of changes in health care, the understanding of key organizational models available to clinicians is critical. Each option has both strengths and weaknesses that only the individual clinician can weigh to choose the best individual model.

Hospital Practice

Hospitals can employ NP's for both inpatient and outpatient services. Inpatient NP services can be billed through Medicare Part B but not Part A. It is risky to bill NP services as "incident to" in a hospital setting and this should be discouraged. Additionally, it is important to be sure a physician is not billing for the same services as the NP on the same date.

Nursing Home Practice

Many NP's find nursing homes to be a great fit for their skills and services. In most cases they are not rushed to see more and more patients and the patients in such facilities lack the preventative care NP's provide. The care of residents in skilled facilities must be under the supervision of a physician who is available in an emergency according to federal law. The federal law also stipulates that at the option of a state, the NP can provide the care if done in collaboration with a physician and not employed by the facility.

Group Practice Without Walls (GPWW)

A model often described as a group practice without walls has emerged as a hybrid between solo and group practice. Members of the practice agree to maintain independent offices yet agree to share key components of the office practice such as billing, management of accounts receivable, and other key fiscal operations. Potential for conflict may exist with less control over daily business functions. The model may exist in different legal forms, to include partnerships, limited liability companies, and professional corporations.

Single Specialty Group Practice

Single specialty group practice is the combination of two or more specialists in the same field to create a group. The benefits of a specialty group practice in addition to the sharing of key office functions as outlined with GPWW include sharing of office space and call coverage. These groups have been very popular in the last several years and many are run by physician practice management companies that can leverage for contracts.

Multi-Specialty Group Practice

A trend in many larger markets has been the consolidation of groups to form large multi-specialty groups. The development of such groups has been driven by the need for greater efficiency, the impact of competitive markets, the effect of large managed care contracts, and the relative stability offered by a larger organization. The majority of multi-specialty groups would be organized as corporations or partnerships.

Solo Practice

Solo practice is traditionally the first choice among physicians but rare for the practicing NP. A solo practice involves operating independently and managing day-to-day operations independent of other providers. Most states require collaboration with a physician for chart review and prescriptive privileges. Hospital privileges and on call coverage may be barriers to such practice.

Evaluating The Right Practice Model For You

Spending time to do a comprehensive evaluation of the available options will result in a more informed decision and hopefully reduce the likelihood of dissatisfaction. The choice you make will likely depend on the level of autonomy you would like to have balanced with the level of risk and stability. Major processes of the decision making process may include talking with colleagues, seeking counsel from an accountant and attorney, and completing a personal inventory or your interests and needs.

Searching

Searching for a nurse practitioner position should not be done in the same manner as looking for a nursing position. You will not find thousands of ads by opening your newspaper, all of them specific to your specialty and location you want to practice. Searching for a nurse practitioner position becomes much more difficult and often times you will have to create one. There are several steps involved in searching for a nurse practitioner position that may make the process a little easier.

Step One: Choose a Geographic Location

The first step in searching for a position is to determine where you are willing to live. There is no sense in searching for a position throughout the country if you have no plans of moving out of the town you currently live in (even if there are no jobs).

Step Two: Choose Your Specialty

The second step in searching is to decide what type of practice setting you hope to work in and the type of specialty you wish to practice. You may think because you are trained in pediatrics for example that you have no choice but to practice in a pediatrician's office or pediatric floor. In reality, there are many more options. Maybe you have a special interest in diabetes care and thus could consider approaching a pediatric endocrinologist in town. Just as well you could approach that large pediatrics group in town and sell the idea of doing the routine follow up care for all the diabetic children in the practice.

Step Three: Look for What's Available

Checking the classified ads has become such an easy task with the world-wide-web. Multiple sites are available that are specific to health care (www.medcareers.com) or even nursing (www.nurse-recruiter.com, www.AANPCareerLink.com) in addition to sites that cover multiple careers (www.monster.com, www.hotjobs.com, www.flipdog.com). Network with faculty and peers who may know of practices searching for a nurse practitioner or at least considering the option.

Step Four: Creating A Position

Often times your best bet is creating a position. This is especially true if you find nothing advertised that fits your niche. This is not at hard as it sounds but requires the ability to sell both yourself and the NP profession. Send out information packets to potential practices. Information packets can include your CV and cover letter along with information about NP's. A nurse practitioner fact sheet that references studies documenting nurse practitioner quality care and high patient satisfaction may be appropriate. The National Association of Pediatric Nurse Associates & Practitioners (NAPNAP) has developed a great brochure for PNP's entitled "The PNP Advantage" that highlights the benefits of hiring a PNP, how to find PNP's and contracting considerations (www.napnap.org). Focus attention on practices that fit your interest and who you know are "busting at the seams" busy. A busy practice may feel the need for another provider but not have the time to look for help. A week or so after you have sent the packet then go visit the medical director to introduce yourself and the benefits of nurse practitioners to a practice and to them in particular. It may help to know their least favorite thing to do in practice (whether it be pelvic exams, taking call, or administrative duties) and offer your expertise in this area.

The Application Process

The application process is often initiated by sending a cover letter and curriculum vitae (CV) in response to an advertisement. Just as a builder needs a hammer and nails to construct a building to sell, you need a CV and cover letter to sell yourself.

The Cover Letter

The cover letter must be of such high quality that the job searcher will both look at your attached CV and call you for an interview. The sole purpose of the cover letter is to get your foot in the door with an interview. The cover letter should be brief (definitely less than 1 page) and professional. The letter should introduce you and your best qualities and relay your interest in the advertised position. The letter should not go into detail but just arouse enough interest in the reader to look at your attached CV. A well-written letter should allow you to do three things:

-Relay the reason for your interest.

-Personalize and target yourself to the particular organization that you are applying to. Don't try to make one cover letter fit all situations.

-Market a specific subset of skills that you have. If you are a new grad then mention the experience you have had as a registered nurse.

There are a few "essentials" of a cover letter. Essential items to include are your contact information, the date, the address of the advertiser, and where you heard of the position being sought. The cover letter should be on good quality bond paper and have a clean, crisp look. There is no reason to add fancy designs, covers or folders. Don't forget to sign the letter and triple check the spelling and grammar for errors. Remember a cover letter alone will not get you a position but will likely be the first thing the employer sees, so make it a good impression.

Resume/Curriculum Vitae

A resume and curriculum vitae (CV) both serve as detailed outlines of your professional experience, training, and credentials. The main difference between a resume and CV are their length. A CV goes into greater depth with regard to publications, conference attendance, and academic achievements. The main components of both include your contact information including all phone numbers, email, address, and fax, your educational background, previous employment, awards and certifications, memberships, community service and you may also include demographic and personal information only if you feel it will benefit you. A resume or CV is often used as a screening device by the employer to determine whom they should interview. Employers usually have an idea of the type of person they are looking for, hoping to find people with a certain educational background or characteristic. Write your resume or CV with this in mind, as just like the cover letter, the goal is to get you an interview. The resume should show that some research has been done to match your skills and with the employer's needs. Successful job hunters convince employers they will become an asset to them.

There are two main types of resumes often labeled chronological and functional. The chronological resume is the most traditional format, which chronologically lists your experiences etc. starting with the most recent. The chronological approach is good for those who's career or educational path have experienced constant growth or for those who have work in progress. The chronological approach is not the best choice for those who have gaps in their career or for those with limited experience. A functional resume emphasizes special skills and accomplishments in order of significance to the position you are applying for. A functional resume stresses what it is you do, rather than what you have done. This type of resume is best for those with limited experiences or training and is not recommended for more professional roles such as NP's. There is no law against combining these two formats as well highlighting both your training and experiences in addition to your specific skill sets, which would be missed in the chronological resume.

The resume should be:

-pleasing to the eye

-honest

-printed on one side of 8 ½ x 11 high-quality paper

-neatly typed on clean neutral color paper with black ink

The resume should not:

-be without a cover letter

-have misspelled words

-include salary needs

-include reasons for leaving a position

-start with the word "Resume"

Professional Portfolio

A professional portfolio is a collection of awards, published papers, projects etc. for the employer to visualize. Many nursing experts recommend using a portfolio. While this may be nice to have it is not necessarily something to bring out right away and often "too much" for the potential employer. A professional portfolio may be particularly helpful when applying for a community oriented position or academic setting where the employer may want to know more about specific accomplishments. The construction of the portfolio may actually be more beneficial than the portfolio itself. Collecting the papers and awards will remind you of accomplishments you have had and thus be ready to market during the interview process.

The Interview Process

The First Interview

After you have submitted your CV and have had an initial telephone interview or discussion, you are ready for your first face-to-face interview. This initial meeting serves mostly as a "get to know" each other meeting. Both you and the interviewer will likely seek to impress one another. Allow your interviewer to get the best of the conversation (if they are willing), talking either about themselves or their practice. Listen attentively as the information they give you will provide you useful information as the interview continues and will tell you a lot about their overall beliefs. If the interviewer does not openly talk about themselves or the practice then ask questions of them along this level. Most people enjoy discussing themselves or their organization if they are proud of it. Ask about their philosophy or style of practicing medicine or the goals of the organization. You are certain to have more questions about how the practice will benefit you (such as how much money you will be making) but hold these back for the second interview. Be attentive as to how your interviewer is presenting themselves as well. Do they make direct eye contact with you? Do they switch subjects or not answer the questions you ask them? Does the interviewer interrupt you when you are talking or do they appear as

Business Essentials for Nurse Practitioners

if they are waiting for you to stop talking, which may be a sign that they do not respect you as a peer.

When the interviewer does ask you questions then take a few seconds to answer instead of blurting out answers. Make sure you think about why they are answering the question before you answer. Stay away from making negative comments or remarks about previous employers or health care situations. If the interview makes such comments and you want to agree that is fine but do not initiate negative discussions. Be sure to know your answers to the most common questions asked in a first interview such as: 1) What are your goals for the next ___# of years?, 2) What is your best quality?, 3) What is your worst quality?, 4) What can you bring to this setting? The key to the first interviewer is to leave a positive impression and to present a win-win situation. Key outcomes your employer can expect are a lightened load from your hiring both clinically and administratively and an increased income for the practice.

Make sure that the interviewer knows that you are interested in the position and excited at the opportunity (if you are). Always follow up after the first interview. Send a thank you letter via the mail the same day of the interview and again let them know that you are interested. In 4-5 days make a telephone call to the person you interviewed. Your persistence will increase the likelihood that you will be asked for a second meeting and shows that you truly are interested.

Key Interviewing Strategies

Show respect to the interviewer. Listen attentively when the interviewer is talking and answer questions honestly.

Be open about your past. Be ready to discuss employment gaps and previous positions that did not work out in a convincing yet honest manner.

Keep the conversation positive at all costs.

Do your homework. Be very familiar with both the practice and the specialty in which you are interviewing. Knowledge is power.

Show your flexibility. As nurses we all have multiple talents. Be sure the interviewer is aware that you can and are willing to do more that just perform direct patient care.

Learn about the interviewer. Don't be afraid to ask questions of the interviewer but try asking questions that interest them. Understanding the person interviewing you will give you a greater chance of having a conversation that leads to highlighting how you can help them.

Money talks, Last. It is not wrong to discuss money during the interview but don't negotiate actual numbers until later interviews. It is generally advised to discuss salary last or wait until a second or third interview even.

"Dress and attitude." Lastly, don't forget the essentials of a good interview including conservative business attire, a positive attitude, and a professional, confident demeanor.

The Second Interview

Before going to the second interview you should plan on doing a little background check on your potential new employer. Find out what you can about the supervising physician's reputation and track record. A small amount of time now can save you from some unpleasant revelations later. Check with your state's medical regulatory board for pending or previous malpractice suits or license suspensions. A few lawsuits are not atypical but if there are a number of suits filed against the same practitioner this may be a red flag. Malpractice insurers are required to report payments made for malpractice claims to the National Practitioner Data Bank 1-800-767-6732.

The second interview will likely be much longer and more in-depth. You may want to ask to observe the physician or practitioner you are interviewing with in action. Observing how the practitioner and office functions can give you a lot of information that would not come about in discussion. The lay out of an office can be quite important as well. If the plan is for you to function with the use of just one exam room it may be difficult for you to see enough patients and thus be profitable. If space is limited then find out how the practice may expand for future growth. The second interview should serve to function as finding out more about the practice, how it functions, and how you will work into the practice. Of course, you will also want to find out more about benefits, hours, and further expectations such as being on call or performing hospital rounds during the second interview.

The interviewer will want to know more about your practice style and how well you will fit into their practice model. Be ready to sell yourself and your profession. Even as a new nurse practitioner you likely have a wealth of experience and expertise as an RN so don't sell yourself short. Emphasize your educational preparation along with your previous experiences in health care even if it is not as an NP. Discuss the health maintenance and prevention approach of nurse practitioners in addition to our diagnosis and treatment ability. Be sure to bring up special interests or skills you bring to the table such as experience performing pap smears or your suturing ability.

Again, don't forget to ask for the job you are interviewing for. You must make sure that the interviewer knows that you are interested in the position and excited at the opportunity. An additional meeting may be appropriate in a more social setting such as over dinner or at one of your homes with your families. How the spouses interrelate with each other is more important than you may think. A working relationship does not require a close social friendship but a nonprofessional level of communication is very helpful. If you are not married then you may not be comfortable with meeting your potential employer alone in this type of social setting. Invite a mutual friend or ask for the practice manager or another important team member of the practice to attend.

Observation Period

Scheduling additional time with one of the practitioners in observation can be very helpful in deciding whether you and the practice are a good fit. If you are not yet out of your training program try to schedule clinical time with the nurse practitioners or physicians in the practice. If you are already out of school then volunteer to spend some unpaid observation time at the practice. Spend as much time possible with the supervising physician. Determining his/her clinical preferences will improve collaboration in the future. The extra time will also give you an opportunity to understand the ground rules when you are working more independently. During this observation period you can learn a lot by asking questions of the nurses and office staff and achieve a sense of whether they are happy with what they are doing and how they are treated by the management team. You can also get a feeling of how receptive the office staff is of having a nurse practitioner provider on board. Leaving a positive impression with the other staff can lean in your favor because they will often give the interviewer their impression of you. Be willing to share personal information as long a you don't think it will hinder you and learn as much personal information of other staff members to achieve a good working relationship before you are even hired.

Evaluating an Offer

A job offer from a private or group practice is very different from that of a hospital as is a nurse practitioner offer is from a registered nursing position. You have more leverage to negotiate salary and benefits because you are now in an income producing position. Evaluating an offer is just like the dating process in many ways. Meeting a potential mate for the first time may have you excited and energetic to get involved but you don't run off and get married on the first date. If you realize a person may be someone you would like to marry you spend time getting to know them recognizing and accepting both the good and bad before you commit to marriage.

Evaluating an Opportunity

☐ How many patient rooms will you be working out of?
☐ Is there space for future growth?
☐ Are there enough support staff to handle your arrival?
☐ Is there a lot of staff turnover?
☐ What is the office overhead?
☐ Is there space in the office for your office/consultation room?
☐ How will the practice promote your arrival?
☐ How many patients do they see and do they plan for you to see?
☐ How is the on-call coverage handled?
☐ How is provider time off handled in the practice?
☐ Will you have access to the practice's profit and loss statements and other financial records to track your productivity?
☐ Is there an orientation period?
☐ How long does it take for a new patient to schedule an appointment?
☐ How long does a patient usually wait to be seen by the provider?
☐ What is the ratio of nurse/provider?
☐ Is the office space owned or leased and for what period?
☐ Are there other duties you will be expected to do besides patient care management such as bring back your own patients?
☐ Can you pursue other opportunities such as research studies?
☐ Is there equipment to perform procedures (rigid sigmoids etc.)?
☐ Do the employees appear happy and satisfied?
☐ Does the supervising physician have time for you to ask questions through the day?

If you find that you and the practice or physician are not a good fit then don't waste each other's time. Write a letter thanking the interviewer for their time and opportunity and then gracefully state that you are not interested in the position. Don't go into detail as to why but rather just mention that it is not a good fit. You will likely meet up with this person again and you do not want to create an uncomfortable situation or relationship.

Making the step toward commitment

If you are offered the position verbally and are definitely interested then accept the position. The details can be worked out later and you will not be bound to a verbal acceptance. A written document will supersede the oral agreement. Write up a letter of intent or have your lawyer do it. A letter of intent can put in writing your requirements for the position or may just put in writing the areas you have already discussed. If the employer finds this acceptable then an employment contract can be drawn out. Read your employment contract or employee manual thoroughly to save yourself from surprises down the road. Most experts even recommend having a lawyer read it over which can save you some time and also allow for some clarification.

Starting Out

Schedule extra time for your new job when you first start. Making a good impression and doing a good job for the patient and your employer take much more time than you ever would have imagined when you were in school. At the start of and end of your day leave some time for interaction with staff members for socializing and "getting to know" those you will be working with. Starting out with good relationships during the "honeymoon" period will pay off greatly later.

While you are still new, use the people who you work with as a valuable information resource. There are all kinds of little things that your employer will not tell you up front but can be very important. To function optimally a practitioner should know what every co-workers responsibilities are and even better how they do them. Take your time with expressing your viewpoint on controversial issues. Most people need to get to know you before accepting new ideas and opinions.

Don't forget to take care of the essentials when starting a new position such as submitting collaborating agreements to your state nursing board and obtaining Medicare, Medicaid and third party insurance carrier billing numbers. If you are the first nurse practitioner in the organization you can expect to do this all yourself. If your aren't the first nurse practitioner in the organization you may still want to oversee this process to be sure it gets done and gets done right.

Chapter 5

Contract Negotiation and Renegotiation

"Never let your collaborating physician know that you know more than they do about a subject"

The Written Agreements

Business in general and the health care industry in particular functions largely through contractual relationships. According to *Webster's Dictionary*, a contract is (1) "a binding agreement between two or more persons or parties," or (2) "a document describing the terms of a contract" (*Merriam-Webster's Collegiate Dictionary*, 1995). Fundamentally a contract is an *agreement*. This chapter like this whole book is not intended as a substitute for legal or other professional advice but should assist the NP in understanding common contracts and issues in relation to them.

Collaborative Practice Agreement (CPA): Written contract defining the joint practice of a nurse practitioner and physician in a collaborative working relationship within the framework of their scopes of practice. CPA's are required in the majority of states for prescriptive authority.

Elements of a good Collaborative Practice Agreement

    A. The manner in which prescription writing and medication dispensing will be handled

    B. Criteria for procedure performance and specialist referrals

    C. Hospital privileges and admission procedures

    D. Policies for chart review and co-signing

    E. Policies for laboratory, radiology and diagnostic testing

    F. Guidelines for patient assignment, triage and on-call

    G. Requirements for co-signatures and chart notations

    H. Coding and billing procedures

    I. Other general medical guidelines and references

Job Description: A job description is a document describing the expectations of any employee for a particular position.

The job description may serve as the basis of performance appraisals by defining the standards of performance related to a particular job. Additionally, the job description can be used to describe a position to a potential job candidate. Duties accounting for more than 5-10% of an employee's time should be included within the job description. The majority of hospitals or large groups who employ nurse practitioners will have a job description in place. In most other cases it will be you researching and providing a job description. Remember the purpose of a job description is to provide written expectations and clarification of duties for a position. Many states require job descriptions for prescriptive authority but beyond this there is no other real legal requirement for a job description. Contact your board of nursing to determine if a job description is a "must have".

Employment contract: Business contract setting forth requirements of both the employee and employer.

An employment contract and a CPA can be one in the same or can be drawn up separately. The CPA will likely contain more clinical issues while the business contract contains employment and financial issues. Employee contracts are beneficial to both the employee and employer. For an employee, the employment contract ensures some measure of job security. For an employer, the contract may afford protection against competition in the future. Employment contracts put important issues to front which otherwise may not be discussed until particular issues arise later. A written employment contract is legally binding to both parties.

Most organizations that have already employed nurse practitioners will have an employment contract to start from. If the employer does not already have an employment contract then it is suggested that you supply one. The employer will almost definitely make changes, but by providing your own you can make sure all the issues are addressed that you feel important. Draft the employment contract in a word processing program or purchase a software program (Quickens Family Lawyer) that will contain all the basics of a contract to start from. When you are finished with the draft then you may want to seek the assistance of a lawyer to go through it with you. By having a contract in draft form you can save a lot of expensive time spent with the lawyer.

Consider an employment agreement similar to a patients medical record, if it is not documented it has not been done or not agreed upon. Verbal agreements do not hold much weight during legal proceedings.

Elements of a Good Employment Contract

Purpose of the Document

Simply describes who are the employee and the employer in the relationship and what the basis of the contract is.

Job Description

Describes the services to be performed. In general this is attached as a separate paper document but referred to as an exhibit.

Hierarchy, department affiliation.

Describes who it is you will be reporting to or who your boss is. At times this may be several individuals such as one person administratively and one person medically.

Duration of employment (Term of the contract)

Describes how long the contract is effective. Some states limit the duration of employment contracts but usually allow at minimum 5 years. There are benefits of having a short-term contract and long-term contract depending on what you feel is most important. A long-term contract may provide you with a feeling of security but a short-term contract may give you more opportunity for renegotiation in the future.

Alteration and updating the contract

Describes how the contract can be editing or renewed.

Licensure requirements, continuing education allowance.

Describes the necessary certifications or licensure requirements that must be met by the employee and how much money they have to use for continuing education.

Compensation

Describes the amount of money the employee will earn for the position agreed upon.

Employee Benefits

Describes the benefits the employer will provide to the employee during the term of the agreement.

Number of hours per week

The employer and employee may have different ideas of how many hours a full-time position requires if not specifically written. Generally speaking a full time NP position will require 40-50 hours of work.

Termination Clause

A termination clause specifies circumstances for firing. An agreement to require termination with cause allows the employer to terminate an NP without notice for unprofessional conduct or moral turpitude, felony conviction, drug or alcohol abuse, or loss of licensure. A termination clause including a without-cause action ("at will") allows either party to end the agreement without specific reason. Termination clauses written with a without-cause action can be written with or without a specified notice time (typically 30-90 days) written in the contract.

Practice Dissolution Clause

A practice dissolution clause states the time period the employee may not work for a competitor of the employer. This clause is often labeled a "Non-compete clause". Typically a time frame such as 2 years is included along with a geographic radius where the employee may not be employed in a given area of practice. The clause in many cases provides for damages if the covenant is breached (usually $50-100,000) and also provides for financial penalties, typically $1,000 per patient solicited and $5,000 per employee solicited.

Performance Evaluation

Determines how often, by what measurements, and in what manner your job performance will be evaluated. A performance evaluation is critical to bringing issues to the forefront. Many times people are reluctant to discuss both the good and bad of a persons performance but without feedback the good may end and the bad will continue because they go unrecognized.

Contract Negotiation

Negotiation is a problem-solving process in which two or more people discuss their needs, interests, and differences in an attempt to reach a joint decision often through bargaining.

Should you hire an attorney?

Nurse practitioners should seek the services of attorneys who are familiar with the laws and legal issues nurse practitioners face. Legal fees may be costly but they will likely be worth it in the long term.

Where do I start?

The most important aspect in contract negotiation is preparation. Proper preparation will allow for optimal negotiation, help you decide what is important to you, and will alleviate some of the anxiety of this stressful situation if you have hard facts and figures.

Step 1

The first step in adequate preparation is prioritizing your specific needs. There are four basic aspects to consider: 1) Compensation, 2) Work hours, 3) Benefits, and 4) The amount of autonomy to practice. The greatest error of many employees is to focus on salary and not consider the rest of the contract. Salary is very dependent on work availability and the geographic area but in most circumstances is the major topic of contract negotiation.

Step 2

Consider the other elements of a contract for negotiation rather than focusing only on salary. Employee benefits may be the best alternative focus of your negotiations. Benefits are quite costly for employers and may nearly equal compensation in some cases. Key benefits to consider include :

Medical and Dental Insurance.

Perhaps the most costly of all benefits, a good medical/dental plan is very important to most individuals and families and will save you a lot of money. The majority of practices/employers will already have a medical/dental plan in place, which may not allow for options. One factor to consider negotiating is payment of premiums and even deductibles by the employer, which can add up to several hundred dollars every month. Recent surveys show 80-90% of midlevel providers receive medical/dental benefits.

Vacation.

Vacation time is another benefit worth negotiating. Establishing a good amount of vacation time early in your career is essential. Employers often don't like extending vacation time later when you become more productive in the practice. Three weeks of vacation has been the average time in salary surveys for the past several years and may be one benefit, which may have slightly decreased, in recent years. Remember time is money and by dividing your salary by 52 will give you a rough idea of what a week of vacation is worth (e.g. $60,000/52wks. = $1154).

Personal and sick time.

These are placed together because they are best placed together in a contract as well. Doing this will allow you to use unused sick time as vacation time. Additionally you can note in the contract that unused sick, personal or vacation time be paid to you in wages at the end of the year or contract period. Do not forget to add in paid holidays.

Malpractice Insurance.

We all need this and a good plan may cost up to several thousand dollars. Include this in your contract with premiums paid by the employer.

Continuing Education.

As professionals continuing education is important and often essential for certification and licensure. Include not only reimbursement for educational fees but also time off and travel expenses. Over 80% of practitioners receive continuing education benefits.

Tuition Reimbursement.

If you are considering furthering your education and/or degree and it will benefit the practice then this may be an important factor as well, considering the rising costs of education. Again, the employer may already have a plan in place for tuition reimbursement, however; a contract allows you to further your benefits. Surveys do show a significant degree of increased wages with higher degrees among nurse practitioners.

Professional Dues.

Professional dues can add up quickly. These can include licensure fees, prescriptive privilege dues, certification renewals, and membership dues to professional organizations.

Automobile, subscriptions, office supplies, pager, cell phones and other practice supplies.

If not in writing it can be an issue. Your idea and the employer's idea of important materials and supplies to practice effectively may differ and become an issue. Putting it in writing gives you and the employer mutually agreed upon guidelines.

Life/Disability Insurance.

Approximately ½ of all practicing NP's have this included in their contract. Yet another key benefit which can be equally important to negotiate in addition to salary.

Retirement.

¾ of practicing NP's have retirement benefits. 401k plans and the like are beginning to be strong recruitment tools. Employer's often place restrictions on enrollment such as continued employment for one year. This can be used as a key negotiating tool along with percentage of employer matching into the plan. Employer matching means that the employer will match your contribution into the plan. 401k plans often limit contributions to 10% of your annual salary and employers can match 0-100% of your contribution.

Financial Incentives

Financial incentives may include reasonable moving expenses, a sign on bonus, a housing allowance, or payment of educational loans.

Productivity Bonus.

Some NP's are against the productivity bonus claiming that it may lead to the practitioner seeing patients as numbers and not individuals. This claim has some merit but not enough to change the recommendation for every NP to have a productivity bonus built into their contract. A productivity bonus rewards the practitioner with a percentage of income when set criteria are met. There are multiple ways productivity bonus' can be written. The majority of bonuses are based on revenue generated or number of patients managed or treated. Most employers are not resistant to productivity bonuses since the bonus will only be paid after certain standards are met (usually meaning you are bringing revenue into the organization. See *Appendix* B for examples of productivity bonuses.

Step 3

Research. Yes, I know you are tired of research but this will give you the important facts & figures you need for negotiating. Start your research on the web by visiting practice organizations such as those listed in the previous chapters that often contain information on negotiation strategies. Web sites such as NP Central (www.nurse.net) and Advance for NP's (www.advanceforNP.com) contain salary and benefit data obtained from surveys of your peers. Local practitioner organizations and practicing NP's may be willing to give you some idea of salary ranges and benefits among area employers for comparison. Look beyond the NP role when researching information. Comparing the costs to employ you versus a new family physician can be very beneficial.

Step 4

Estimate your worth. Estimating your worth includes documenting and discussing your education and professional experience and perhaps estimating your potential generated income into the practice or organization. Several simple equations exist which can give you a good idea of the amount of income you can generate into a practice (see appendix A).

Step 5

Let the negotiating begin. This step will often make you a little diaphoretic. Following the above steps first will help to strengthen your confidence, alleviate some anxiety and allow you to remember what is important to you. When the discussion begins follow these general guidelines:

Determine your minimum salary and benefits ahead of time (do not tell them what this is).

Do not be the first to bring up salary. If asked, make statements to put it back on their shoulders (e.g. I am much more interested in the position as NP here at _____ then I am in the initial offer. I will consider any reasonable offer. You are in a better position to know how much I am worth to you than I am.)

Remember you are on their side, and make certain they know this. An optimal employer/employee relationship will be a win/win situation meaning you will both benefit from the relationship.

Do not dominate the discussion. Be assertive but not aggressive.

Step 6

Put it in writing. Remember if it is not written it is not legally binding. Do not be the only person to review it. People by nature are more precise when writing than when speaking probably because most of us are better readers than listeners. The act of writing out the agreement also serves to improve communication. Make 3-4 originals of each document so that copies can be provided to the practice, the practitioner, the lawyer, and possibly the board of nursing or medicine.

Step 7

Celebrate. Celebrate your new position, new contract, and new partnership. Take your employer and his/her family out to dinner or celebrate on your own.

Salary

Although I believe you should not focus all your efforts on salary during negotiating it still remains likely the most important aspect of employment. Only your salary will pay the mortgage and supermarket bills. Fortunately, the last several years have brought in an average increase of five thousand dollars per year. The increase is quite good when compared to that of physicians salary increases which have been sparing in recent years. Currently, the average nurse practitioner salary is just over $63,000 per year and hourly rate approximately $33.00/hour. There is a lot of variation however and some NP's (usually not in family practice) are making over $150,000 where others barely reach that of an average RN ($38,000).

Multiple factors influence salary including practice setting, geographic area, degree, and unfortunately to this day gender. The gender gap is narrowing in our field however and the gap may be partly due to the low representation of men in the profession. Particular practice settings such as emergency care centers and home health agencies are atop the salary list while public health and by no surprise academia round out the bottom. Nurse practitioners with higher degrees will be happy to know that additional education correlates with salary increases. A doctorate prepared NP can expect to make close to $5,000 more than their Master's prepared counterparts. A few years experience can also add a few thousand dollars onto your salary. The geographic region where you practice may affect your salary as well. The highest paid regions are of course those regions that have more difficulty attracting nurse practitioners such as Alaska and Washington. Areas with an abundance of NP's and NP programs will see lower salary ranges. You will also find higher salaries in more urban versus rural settings in most cases. Most experts agree that there will not likely be significant salary gains in the next several years related to such an extensive focus on cost cutting in health care.

NP's are underpaid in comparison to their physician counterparts. The cost of providing care to a patient remains the same whether the patient is seen by an NP or a physician. The average salary for a primary care physician ranges from $120-150,000 while a primary care NP can expect less than $65,000. This discrepancy equals extra income for the practice. The majority of NP's are paid guaranteed salaries which may provide security but in most circumstances results in a lower income. Implementing a productivity based compensation method can bring a win-win situation to the NP and her employer.

NP Salaries by Setting	
Family practice	62,000
Pediatrics	62,000
Internal medicine	62,000
Emergency care	77,000
Independent practice	80,000
Home health	75,000
Academic	58,000
Public health	56,000

Physician Salaries by Specialty	
Family practice	150,000
Pediatrics	148,000
Internal medicine	148,000
Emergency care	200,000
Cardiology	290,000
Geriatrics	150,000
Neurology	180,000
Orthopedic surgery	340,000
Urgent care	160,000
Anesthesiology	260,000

Salaries of Other Health Care Workers	
Pharmacist	77,000
Physician Assistant	71,000
Social Worker	50,000

Compensation Programs/Productivity Formulas

Although salary is a sensitive subject for most nurse practitioners (NP) it is certainly an important issue both personally and for the profession. NP's compensation methods vary greatly, from guaranteed salaries, to productivity driven formulas, and even hourly wages. Generally, while a guaranteed salary may bring you comfort in security, practitioners with productivity-based salaries have higher incomes. Productivity is income based on objective or at times subjective factors such as number of patients seen, hours worked, total charges, net income, other duties such as management activities, or patient satisfaction scores. If productivity income is based on collections, which most are, one must consider the net to expense ratio. Most primary care practices have a ratio of 50:50 to 70:30. Expenses which factor in to NP compensation include office rent, utilities, salaries and benefits to support staff, medical and office supplies, insurance, and other expenses that come with running a medical practice. Many NP's are unaware of their "Contribution Margin" which is a business term defined as the revenue generated by a provide minus the cost attributed to their efforts (or costs the practice would not have incurred without the provider). Additional factors to consider when determining NP compensation include physician consultation that can be estimated at 5-15% of net income and the risk of doing business involved by the employer also estimated at 5-15%.

Productivity compensation methods encourage higher productivity, than the guaranteed salary but can add to the complexity of determining compensation. Specific circumstances to keep in mind before leaning toward a productivity compensation method include exactly how many patients you would like to see a day, the payer mix you serve, and the collection rate of the practice. Managed care, Medicare, and Medicaid patients tend to be more time consuming and produce less income. If you plan on minimizing the number of patients you see each day (such as <15) you may be better off with a simple guaranteed salary. A good collection rate is at least 90% of billed charges considering your rates are reasonable. Newer NP's should not expect to benefit greatly from a productivity based compensation in their first year of practice but it can still pay off in the long run if your willing to sacrifice early on.

A good idea may be to attach a productivity bonus to your guaranteed salary contract. This means you can have a set salary and receive additional compensation when certain criteria are met. The bonus can be an increase in base salary when you reach an average number of patients seen daily, a percentage of charges in excess of the income that meets your salary needs, or an overall percentage of net income generated. Don't forget other sources of income NP's can generate such as consulting work, research opportunities, and other business opportunities.

Keys in Determining Productivity Compensation and Bonuses:

-Use real number when determining revenues and put in writing how this information will be gathered.

-Make sure you have access to your productivity numbers or develop a way you can do this yourself. You need to know what your doing for the practice financially.

-Keep it simple. Sophisticated compensation methods may lead to disagreement. Focus on just one or two incentive methods rather than complicating things with several which take time and money to calculate.

-Become familiar with how you will function in the practice and how this will affect the productivity numbers. Will you be bringing your own patients back, taking their vital signs, and discharging them on your own or will you have assistants to help with the tasks you need not perform.

-Be familiar with the functioning of the "back office". Know who sets up the fee schedules with the practice's major payers, how they respond to denied claims and how they determine the charges.

Renegotiating

Contract renegotiating is not all that different from negotiating your first contract. You still do not want to go into it unprepared. You need to put forth a lot more effort than walking into your physician or practice manager's office and asking for a raise. The steps are similar for renegotiating but at this point you should have a lot more information at your hands.

Step 1

Prioritize your needs. Does your focus remain the same or are you now searching for more time off as opposed to a higher salary.

Step 2

Consider other benefits which interest you rather than focusing on salary. A more flexible schedule, less work hours, extra vacation time, or additional continuing education benefits are all possible requests you can make in lieu of a salary increase. This may be the opportunity to discuss a productivity bonus now that you are likely bringing income into the practice.

Step 3

Research. Do you homework on average salary increases in the area and around the country. Be familiar with your generated income into the practice.

Step 4

Estimate you're worth using *appendix A* or income sheets from the previous year. Reasonably determine what percentage of your generated income the practice should pay you. Your stress level will go down if you have a good set of figures to work with.

Step 5

Set up an appropriate time with your employer to discuss your contract demands. It is important to have adequate time to focus attention to the topic at hand. Keep a good attitude during your meeting and look toward creating a "win-win" situation.

Step 6

Put it in writing with either an addendum to your old contract or with a whole new contract.

Successful Negotiation Tips

-Do your research and always be prepared.

-Have a back-up plan. If the employer does not meet your expectations in one category (salary) then ask for more in another (increased vacation).

-Make sure you talk to the person who is making the decisions.

-Speak with confidence and professionalism.

-Don't blame or accuse anyone for anything.

-Be both objective and reasonable.

Chapter 6

Reimbursement of NP's

"Without reimbursement a job becomes volunteer work"

Achieving adequate reimbursement for NP's has been quite costly and difficult. However challenging reimbursement may be it remains one of the key components of justifying Nurse Practitioner existence. As a registered nurse, NP's are well aware how the lack of direct reimbursement negatively influences our value as a profession. Direct reimbursement not only influences professional value but also allows for the tracking of quality of care measure via payers databases.

Government Programs

The Health Care Financing Administration (HCFA) has recently been renamed the Centers for Medicare and Medicaid Services (CMS). The name change according to the DHHS is symbolic of a new focus for the agency, which is directed to being more responsive to the needs of providers and beneficiaries. 1-800-Medicare has also been enhanced to provide 24-7 service and information. CMS has been divided into three separate centers: the Center for Beneficiary Choices, the Center for Medicare Management, and the Center for Medical and State Operations.

Medicare

The Medicare program is in place to provide basic health insurance coverage to the majority of Americans 65 years or older as well as people who are medically disabled or who have end-stage renal disease. Medicare is a federally funded program created with the Social Security Act of 1965 and expanded in 1972 and 1973. Medicare is the largest source of health care funding in the United States at this time. In 1999, close to 39 ½ million beneficiaries were enrolled in the program, which amounted to over $206 billion in nationwide Medicare benefit payments. Medicare is divided into two separate programs, Part A and Part B. Part A, is usually provided automatically to people aged 65 and older and to most disabled people. It provides inpatient hospital coverage and includes coverage for skilled nursing services, home health, and hospice care. Part B, which is supplementary, pays particular costs of services provided in an outpatient environment including physicians visits, outpatient hospital services, durable medical equipment (DME) and other services not covered by Part A. Part B is subject to monthly premium payments by beneficiaries.

Nurse practitioners can bill Medicare directly for services, but receive only 85% of the physician fee schedule. Nurse practitioners were given the right to bill Medicare directly in 1998 with the Public Law 105-33. The new law grants payment to NP's regardless of geographic area. Previously, NP's had to bill "incident to" physicians services unless they were distinguished as serving in a rural clinic meeting federal guidelines.

Obtaining a Medicare number has become easier with documents from the CMS available online (www.hcfa.gov). The application may be long and tedious but asks for basic information regarding your credentials and information about your practice. Expect approval to take beyond a month and maybe two. Medicare will provide you with both a provider identification number (PIN) and a unique physician identification number (UPIN). The PIN number is used for claims submission and is unique to each site where you practice. The UPIN number is used when ordering durable medical equipment and in some cases when referring to a specialist or other medical service. Nurse practitioners applying to Medicare must hold a national certification and by 2003 will also need to have a Master's degree. Nurse practitioners holding a Medicare number before 2003 will be "grand fathered" into the system. A recent 5.4 percent cut in provider reimbursement for 2002 may lead to some physicians limiting their acceptance of patients on Medicare. Decisions such as this may create a greater need and opportunity for NP's to provide care to these clients.

Medicaid

Medicaid (Title XIX of Social Security Act) was initiated by the government to provide health care insurance coverage for individuals in financial need. The federal and state government funds Medicaid. Medicaid is controlled mostly by the state but under federal guidelines. Medicaid was initially derived to only cover very-low income persons and for the most part continues this way. Medicaid is also restricted to families with children, women who are pregnant, or persons who are aged, or disabled. The range of services of the Medicaid program includes outpatient and inpatient acute care, diagnostic studies, practitioner services, home health care under certain guidelines, many screening services, and extended nursing care for persons over the age of 21. States often provide Medicaid services within a chosen statewide insurance program. The Medicaid program is overseen by the CMS. Certified FNP's and PNP's are covered under Medicaid effective with The Budget Reconciliation Act of 1989 but must apply for a provider number. NP's are reimbursed 100% of what physicians would be paid for the same services. Applications can be obtained from your state Medicaid program.

Federal reimbursement programs are always secondary to other insurance carriers. This means that Medicare and Medicaid will only be billed charges not covered by the patients other insurance carrier(s) it there is one. Medicaid is always billed secondary to Medicare. Providers must accept Medicaid payment as payment in full for services rendered. A personal identification number (PIN) is used to bill for services.

CHAMPUS/FEHBP

CHAMPUS or The Civilian Health and Medical Program of the U.S. is an insurance program that primarily covers military and their family members. NP's are

covered under this program as well as FEHBP. FEHBP
(Federal Employees Health Benefit Program) provides
health benefits to federal employees.

"Incident to" billing

"Incident to" billing is described as the billing of NP
services incident to or under the direction of a
physician. Certain requirements must be met to bill
"incident to" a physician including but not limited to:

-The NP must be employed or leased by the physician
they are billing "incident to".

-The NP must only be providing follow-up care.

-The physician must be present in "the office suite".
The "office suite" has yet to be specifically defined but
it is generally accepted that the physician need not be
in the patient room. If a physician is not on site than
you cannot use "incident to" billing.

-If you are making a new diagnosis you cannot use
"incident to" billing.

-If you are making a medication adjustment then you
cannot use "incident to" billing.

-If the physician has never seen the patient you cannot
bill "incident to."

-Additionally, the service cannot be provided in a
hospital inpatient setting.

"Incident to" billing limits the autonomy of the NP.
Then why are many practices billing "incident to"?
"Incident to" billing allows for 100% reimbursement of
the physician rate while billing directly under the NP

provides only 85% reimbursement of the physician rate. Billing "incident to" when the service you provide is not incident to the physician is considered Medicare fraud. Remember there is also no such thing as billing "incident to" in a hospital inpatient setting.

The Nurse Practitioner and practice manager have two options when billing Medicare: 1) Bill all services by the NP under his/her own Medicare provider number. This decreases the likelihood of fraud but automatically accepts 85% reimbursement of the physician rate on all cases. 2) Billing services "incident to" in cases where services are incident to the physician and billing those services which are not incident to the physician under the NP's provider number. This method increases the risk for fraud to occur but allows some of the visits to be reimbursed at 100% the physician rate. The choice is yours and your practice managers to make. Certainly, billing "incident to" can increase reimbursement rates but if there is not a good system in place to make sure that "incident to" really is "incident to" then you may be better off always billing under your number. Private insurance may not have guidelines for the "incident to" billing method, but you will want to read over each contract.

Private Health Insurance

Despite many recent changes private insurance organizations continue to provide the major source of health care funding in America. The majority of large employers offer health insurance as a benefit to their employees through private insurance companies. There are well over 1000 private insurance companies in the United States today. Fee for service is rapidly being replaced by managed care, which increases the financial risk of health care providers.

Indemnity Insurance

The more traditional form of private health insurance companies, indemnity plans pay providers on "fee for service" basis. Health care services are generally paid on a "usual and customary" basis where certain procedures or visits are paid a set fee that is often based on an average charge in the area for the same service. The charge submitted by the provider really does not matter because they will pay the same standard fee no matter what price are charging. The patient can be charged the reminder of the cost but many times the practice will just accept what the indemnity plan pays. Indemnity plans are not involved in the delivery of care.

Managed Care Organizations (MCO's)

Managed care consists of the integration of delivery and financing of health care. Health plans such as HMO's and PPO's provide members prepaid access to health care at a lower cost. In theory, managed care is designed to foster the effective and appropriate monitoring of a populations health.

PPO's

Preferred provider organizations (PPO's) attempt to provide health care at a lower cost to beneficiaries (those paying for the plan) by giving lower insurance premiums. A PPO is a form of MCO plan that uses a provider network to render care. Providers who choose to be and are accepted into the plan are paid discounted rates. Providers may choose to join such a plan in order to increase their volume of patients offsetting the discounted rates. The higher degree of flexibility of PPO's has put them into the majority of MCO's.

HMO's

A health maintenance organization (HMO) is a form of MCO that offers health care to participating members for a fixed and prepaid amount or premium with the contract that members must see networked providers. Providers who choose to be a networked or participating provider receive prepaid payments to care for a group of enrolled patients for a specific range of comprehensive services. The provider thus shares some of the risk of the HMO hoping their group of patients remain healthy or use less health care services. Enrollees are usually assigned to receive health care services from a primary care provider.

EPO's

Exclusive provider organizations (EPO's) limit their members to only receive health care from its network of providers. Care received outside of the network is not covered except in some emergency situations.

MSO

A managed services organization (MSO) is an organization that performs the enrollment, claims processing and management services for enrolled health plans.

MCO's premiums have been escalating rapidly in the last few years as the public is expressing desire for less restrictive MCO's such as PPO's. It is because the insured person has only a small amount of financial burden associated with their health-care, they have not felt the need to pressure insurance companies further to keep rates low.

Managed Care Terms

Capitation: the prepayment for health care services to providers on a per member basis occurring most often on a monthly basis. No matter what the costs incurred in caring for the members.

Co-payment: the amount of the medical expense paid by the insured out of pocket at the time of the visit.

Coinsurance: the amount paid by the insurer when a plan limits its coverage by a percentage. 80 percent is often the limited amount leaving 20 percent to be paid by the insured

A deductible is the amount the insured must pay "out of pocket" before any insurance coverage begins to apply. Deductibles often range from $100 to $2000.

Contracting with MCO's

Managed care has penetrated the majority of the United States overseeing the health care services for a large number of Americans. Contracting with MCO's has become more a necessity than a choice for providers of health care. The historical goal of MCO's to provide access to high quality care has been clouded according to many experts by its goal of providing cost-effective care. Before joining MCO's the NP must determine whether the negotiated rates are worth the risks associated with capitation.

Essential steps to take before signing as an MCO provider include:

-Obtain specific costing data and statistical information in order to make an informed decision.

-Negotiate rates fairly.

-Clarify ambiguous data and contract details.

-Seek a Win-Win situation.

-Read the contract in its entirety.

-Be sure your name will be on the directory and not listed under your collaborating physicians name.

Although a minority, some MCO's choose not to credential NP's, however, this is more likely attributed to a low number of actual applicants. A few health insurers argue that they can't impanel NP's because NP's are not allowed to practice independently. They do not understand the differences between independent practice versus collaboration mandates. MCO reimbursement to NP's is often done through a supervising or collaborating physician making NP's invisible in the system. If you are providing services under your collaborating physicians identification then seek to add MCO contract language that states services rendered may be provided by the physicians or NP.

The Managed Care Trend

Consumer demand is shifting back away from capitated systems where participants have less of a choice back to fee-for-service organizations which now offer discounted services. The growth of MCO's has recently flattened meaning employers are having to pay higher rates during an economic downswing. It is expected that eventually employers will shift these costs to the employee who will again search for some form of change.

Chapter 7

Marketing You and The Practice

"If customers are not coming to see you then go to them"

Many practitioners falsely assume that once they open
their doors or start their new position the patients will
start streaming in, after all everyone will become ill at
some point in time. Many others do not consider
marketing to be an important ingredient in a medical
practice or feel as though they are unable to market
their practice. Marketing becomes even more important
for the NP provider who the public is less familiar with
than the physician.

The 4 P's of Marketing

Product, Price, Place, and Promotion have long been the
standard elements in any marketing course or lecture
series but continue to be a good starting ground. The
first step in any marketing plan should be to establish
the 4 P's of your practice. It is often best to establish
your 4 P's through the eyes of your patient or guest to
your practice.

The first P stands for *product*. The NP's product is the
clinical service they provide to the patient. Right? Well
yes, but try to think of your product as "health and
wellness". In order to compete in health care NP's must
differentiate their product by communicating the
benefits of NP care. A well-known benefit of NP care is
their focus on the promotion of health and wellness as
opposed to physicians who often focus on the treatment
of disease and illness. Additionally, by developing a
niche you can further differentiate your services (such
as combining both traditional and non-traditional
medicine). *Price*, the second P, not only deals with the
cost of services but also proper utilization of health care
services and total cost effectiveness. Compare your
price to your competitors and if your price is lower then
this should be well known. The third P is *place* or the
geographic and physical structure of where you practice.
The right location of a practice can play a big role in

your popularity among potential clients. Before opening a new office or moving to a location the site should be investigated thoroughly. Key factors in choosing a site include the location of competitors, the location of the population you are hoping to serve, office availability, accessibility, and the "not to forget" aesthetics of the place. *Promotion* the fourth and last P is the ability to communicate your message to potential clients. Through the use of promotional modes such as advertisements, word of mouth testimonials, community presentations, etc. the goal is to increase the community awareness of your practice. The biggest mistake NP's make in marketing is not placing enough effort and money into their promotional efforts.

Tracking Return on Investment

To accurately identify both winning and losing marketing efforts it is essential to establish a tracking program. A simple tracking program will do. The key ingredient in a marketing tracking program is to document how new patients become familiar with you and your practice. The perfect time for this to occur is when the patient is scheduling their first visit or during their first visit. Do not let a new patient leave your office after the first visit without having asked how they came to you. After developing an adequate tracking plan you can use the results to track return on investment (ROI). Return on investment simply stated is the amount of money returned to you in comparison to the amount of money you put forth in the endeavor. For, example if you paid $200 for an advertisement that resulted in 10 new patients the ROI would be very good. Considering that each new patient to a primary care setting will generate at least $20-$30 at the initial visit and perhaps several thousand dollars over time. Tracking ROI will allow you to accurately identify good and poor marketing strategies. This information will tell you where to put your marketing money and effort.

Seven Simple and Economical Marketing Efforts to Bring in New Patients and Keep Existing Patients

1. Ask your patients for referrals

At first this will be very uncomfortable to do. However, don't give up. Once you start and stay with it the more comfortable it will be. Start with your patients who come in overjoyed with what you have done for them. If they come in not satisfied or with unresolved symptoms, don't ask them. When you find that delighted patient say something such as "Well I am glad we have things well controlled now, you know if you know of anyone else with similar problems send them in, I'd love to help them as well". This is only a few seconds of conversation but can do a great deal with the amount of ease they feel with sending you someone. This small step will undoubtedly increase your number of word-of-mouth referrals by over 15 percent.

2. Recognize every patient referral

Thank your patients, collogues, and friends with every referral they give you. Recognizing each referral they give will actually motivate them to send you more. Not recognizing them will make them stop referring to you because they will feel as though you don't need their help or are not thankful of the business. You can thank them in several ways but you should always thank them in person either at their next visit or with a phone call. The phone call should ideally occur soon after the referral comes in. Follow up your personal thank you with a quick *handwritten* card or small gift. You may want to save the gift giving for the point where they have sent you 2 or more referrals. You should develop a list of those who have referred to you and how many referrals they have sent you. Gradually increase the value of the gifts you give to them with each referral they send you. For example after receiving 3 referrals from the same person send them a small useful gift such as a nice letter opener with your name on it. Stay away from flowers and candy that have no lasting value. When they send you the 4th or 5th referral then send something with value such as a gift certificate to a fine restaurant. If someone goes beyond this then don't be afraid to spend $50-$100 on concert tickets or perhaps a large plant for their home or office. All of this may sound expensive but one new patient who stays with your practice can generate greater than $7,000 while in your practice.

3. Develop a new patient orientation mailing

Send your scheduled new patients a kit containing information about your practice reinforcing the need to keep their appointment with you and making them aware of the services you offer. The kit should contain at minimum a welcome letter but can also include a brochure, business card, map to the office, marketing resume, and journal or newspaper articles about your practice. Have the front office staff put these together and mail one out every time a new patient is scheduled. This simple step will decrease your new patient no-shows and will make them more familiar and comfortable with you at their first visit.

4. Utilize a Marketing Resume

A marketing resume is quite different from a traditional resume or curriculum vitae. A marketing resume is intended to promote you to customers that are unfamiliar with you. A marketing resume should include some things traditional resumes do not such as your picture and maybe a discussion about your hobbies and family if you are comfortable with this. This information automatically makes you more personable to your patients. A marketing resume also includes the traditional information such as your training, certifications, published literature, research interests, awards, community projects etc. Remember when writing a marketing resume that you are not speaking to an employer but instead a future customer. For an example see *Appendix N*. The marketing resume can be utilized in the following ways: a) included in your new patient mailing, b) handed to the new patient by the front office staff before the patient is brought back to see you, c) handed out during lectures or at symposiums and/or d) left out in your waiting room lobby. The simple steps in developing and using a marketing resume will increase your credibility and likeability with your patients.

5. Develop a Recall System

A recall system is set up to remind your patients to return for their follow-up visits. An adequate recall system actually needs to involve 5 key steps. The first step will be the discussion you have with the patient during the visit. This involves explaining to the patient the importance of the next follow up visit ("It is important for you to be seen in 6 months so that we can assure you are on the correct dose of the medication"). The second step is having the front office staff help the patient set up their next appointment while they are paying their co-pay or going through the discharge process in your office. Letting them leave without setting an appointment will reduce the likelihood of a timely follow-up. Step three involves a reminder postcard mailed at least a week in advance of the appointment. This step can be done by hand or via a software system. The fourth step consists of a telephone call just one to two days in advance of the appointment by your office staff or by an electronic system (www.prominders.com). Not everyone is good at keeping an appointment book and this step can cut your no shows in half. Most patients at this point are assured to show up at their visit or at least will reschedule their appointment. The fifth and last step will reach those who have missed their follow-up visit or have canceled and not rescheduled. Many of these patients may feel the appointment is not necessary or feel they don't have time for the visit. The art of bringing this patient back in to see you lies in stressing the importance of the visit. For example, a patient with hyperlipidemia fails to follow-up at their requested 6-month visit. A personally signed letter is sent stressing the importance of the visit ("It is important for us to measure liver function tests to assess for potential side effects from your medication") a week or two after their appointment was due. This step can be repeated in another 1-2 months if the patient continues to not make it in. You may also decide to hold refills on their medications until they make their return visit and a note in the letter explaining the risks of side effects without proper monitoring.

6. Develop Professional Stationary

Whatever the size of your practice a good stationary system can make your practice seem larger. Your stationary should communicate your services and/or benefits of your practice to both your patient and referrers. Components of a stationary system at minimum should include business cards, envelopes, and letterhead. Add a personal logo to your stationary to establish a brand for your practice. A brand gives your practice a trademark or a key identifier. Utilize your stationary with all correspondence including recall letters, referral letters, and letters to friends or collogues. The stationary will reinforce the benefits of your practice with each piece of stationary they receive from you. Many marketing and advertising firms can assist with the development of your stationary (www.vistaprint.com). Business cards are cheap so use them every chance you get: hand them to all new patients, leave them laying out after a lecture given by you, hand them out to everyone you meet, and put them on bulletin boards at your church and gym.

7. Develop Referral Relationships with Collogues

Nurse Practitioners do not do this nearly as well as physicians or other professionals. Send referrals to your NP peers who may specialize in another area of practice and in turn they will likely do the same. Relationships such as this are a win-win-win situation. The patient benefits from receiving specialized care and both practitioners benefit from the increase in business. This also works with friends who are not NP's such as a friend who may own a vitamin and herbal shop or an acquaintance who is a chiropractor. An additional strategy may be to advertise each other's products or services in your waiting room, on your web site, or even in a mailing.

And a few more advanced steps

Build a Web Site

Developing a web site can be simpler than you think with some sites offering to build your site for free in turn for using their hosting services. Hosting is the process of keeping your web site active on the World Wide Web. Keep your site simple with general information about your practice such as location, specialty and philosophy together with links to sites you trust for patients to find accurate information on varying illnesses or prevention. This is another place where you can mention or advertise the business of a collogue in return for their advertising your practice on their site. Put your web site address on your business cards, stationary and all of your advertising material. A web site can be easier to remember than a phone number for a potential client when they are looking to find you at a later date. Remember this when you are choosing your web address so that you keep it simple and easy to remember.

Develop a Practice Brochure

Again you can do this yourself or higher an expert. A practice brochure is a somewhat flashy marketing tool that should be designed for the client in mind. Appealing pictures and great testimonial statements should take much of the space rather than general information. The practice brochure should convince the reader they need to come see you. Your practice brochure can be used in direct mailings, left out during community presentations, given to key referrers, and left in your lobby for current patients to take home.

Have the Biggest Yellow Page Advertisement

This is one case where bigger is definitely better. A good yellow page ad can be the most productive marketing effort you have. Clients will naturally gravitate towards the largest ad assuming the company with the biggest ad is the largest and best in its class. You can take advantage of this even if you aren't the largest in town but it will cost you. Yellow page ads are quite expensive but are reaching a large target audience. Yellow page ads should be constructed to be fairly simple yet get the message across.

News Ads

News ads can also be fairly expensive to run but can have a good return on investment if you are in need of new patients. Remember the audience you will reach with a newsprint ad will generally be over the age of 30, well educated and middle to upper socioeconomic class. Your ad should be placed in the section more particular to your clientele. For example, if you have an ob-gyn practice then you are better off placing your ad in the leisure and food section rather than in the sports section. A newsprint ad should be similar to a phonebook ad with a simple nature but addressing the benefits of your practice.

Press Release

A press release is one way to get free coverage in the newspaper. Writing a press release does not guarantee that you will get coverage but it is well worth the effort. Press releases can be written about an aspect of your practice or a new medical treatment or discovery you are interested in. An article in the newspaper mentioning your name or practice can often bring in even more patients than an advertisement. People tend to put more trust into an article than that of an advertisement. *See Appendix G.*

Radio and Television Ads

These are both very expensive and usually will result in poor return on investment. I would stay away from this type of advertising unless you come across a great deal. However, if you are asked to be interviewed on a talk show or by a news crew, jump at the opportunity.

Start a Practice Newsletter

More time consuming than expensive, a practice newsletter can act as a marketing tool as well as an educational tool for your patients. Write reviews on common illnesses such as those you have just read about in your latest journal. Include in the newsletter any new services or changes within your practice. Sent out quarterly to your patients they are reminded of your services and may pass it on to friends and family.

The "Double Hit" Phenomenon

A potential client is more prone to make a decision to come to your practice if they have seen or heard of your practice in more than one way. Thus, it is important to use more than just one avenue for marketing your practice. For instance, you may meet a person at an event and hand them your business card with your web site listed conveniently on the front. Later, while surfing the web they make a visit to your site where they see you specialize in an area they could use help with.

Developing a Marketing Plan

After reading through this chapter and maybe a few other sources on marketing develop your own marketing plan. There are many software programs to help you do this (Microsoft Small Business Software) and make it quite easy.

Chapter 8

The Basics of Coding and Billing

"When the administrators talk about improving productivity, they are never talking about themselves."

It is recommended that you have both a CPT® and ICD-9 coding book available to reference while reading this chapter.

Coding is the term used to describe the process of assigning identifying codes to the services and procedures we perform and the diagnosis we use to describe symptoms or illness. The American Medical Association developed the CPT® (Current Procedural Terminology) codes, which provide a recognized language describing the medical, surgical, and diagnostic services physicians and nurse practitioners provide. The Medicare Catastrophic Coverage Act of 1988 mandated the use of ICD-9-CM (International Classification of Diseases, 9th revision, Clinical Modification) codes to describe diagnosed illness, symptoms, or health screening. Coding is now the universal language in billing for medical services for the physician and nurse practitioner as well. Many nurse practitioners would like to see our own set of codes based more on the preventative services nurse practitioners provide. In reality, however, for now we will have to stick to the universal codes that lead to reimbursement.

ICD-9 Coding (Diagnosis Codes)

The ICD-9 codes were first written by the World Health Organization to classify morbidity and mortality information. The codes were expanded for use in the hospital setting and now the U.S. Department of Health and Human Services and the Centers for Medicare and Medicaid Services (CMS) provides a version ICD-9-CM that is more precise. The ICD-9-CM version is used in most clinical settings and is updated every October by the CMS. The ICD-9 codes classify and arrange diseases and injuries into grouped categories. The ICD-9 codes are numerical numbers that are 3-5 digits in length. The codes are usually followed by a description of the code but insurance companies often just look at the number. The ICD-9 codes are well recognized by third party payers including Medicaid and Medicare. In fact, the codes must be used in most situations in order for claims to be accepted. Several publishers put out a listing of the updated codes annually (www.medicalbookstore.com) and it is essential for every office to have at least one copy of these. You should have a copy for yourself and be well familiar with how to look up codes and whether a 3,4, or 5-digit code is required. Many payers are now requiring certain ICD-9 codes be listed for the ordering (or at least payment) of particular diagnostic testing.

The process of coding has become more and more difficult and confusing since there are more and more diseases and illnesses that we are discovering or naming. Medical coding and billing has become a specialty of its own and a specialty certification is even offered. The difficulty in staying abreast of coding and billing issues is that they are ever-changing and soon there will be ICD-10 codes to relearn. You can hire the best of coders but the truth is that the provider is always responsible for the coding in legal matters. All providers should have a good working knowledge of the coding system and if you have someone else doing your coding you should be familiar with what they are doing.

Understanding the Numbers

The ICD-9 codes are first classified into sections of diseases and injuries by groups of the first 3 digits. There are seventeen different groups plus two supplementary groups (V and E codes).

001-139	Infectious and Parasitic Diseases
140-239	Neoplasms
240-279	Endocrine, Nutritional, Metabolic Diseases and Immunity Disorders
280-289	Blood Diseases
290-318	Mental Disorders
320-389	Nervous System Diseases
390-459	Circulatory System Diseases
460-519	Respiratory System Diseases
520-579	Digestive System Diseases
580-629	Genitourinary System Diseases

630-676	Complication of Pregnancy, Childbirth, and Puerperium
680-709	Skin Diseases
710-739	Musculoskeletal and Connective Tissue Diseases
740-759	Congenital Anomalies
760-779	Perinatal Period Conditions
780-799	Signs, Symptoms, and Ill Defined Conditions
V Codes	Factors Influencing Health Status
E Codes	External Causes of Poisoning and Injury

Each disease then has its own three-digit number, which falls within the number of its classified group.

For example the number 493 describes *Asthma*. As you can see it falls within the group of numbers describing diseases of the Respiratory system.

A fourth digit is then added in some cases to describe the disease further or to add clinical detail.

For example 493.1 describes *Intrinsic Asthma*.

An added fifth digit sub-classifies the condition even further.

For example 493.12 describes *Intrinsic Asthma with acute exacerbation.*

Not all codes have a fifth digit or even a fourth digit but if you can sub-classify the disease then you should. In some circumstances Medicare will not allow just a 3-digit code (e.g. 492 *Emphysema*) unless a fourth digit is added to further classify the condition (e.g. 492.8 *Emphysema obstructive*). Some ICD-9 publications will make this simple by color-coding the codes telling you whether a forth or fifth digit is required. For example the code 493 may be in the color red indicating adding a fourth digit is required. The codes may also contain some use of abbreviations you may need to become familiar with (e.g. *NOS* stands for Not Otherwise Specified).

When you go to look up a code you can look it up alphabetically by the conditions name (*Asthma*) or you can look under the group (Diseases of the Respiratory System) that the diagnosis would fall under if you are unsure of the name. If you are certain of the disease you are working with then you should use the code for this condition (e.g. 493.1 *Intrinsic Asthma*) but if you do not have a high level of certainty as to the condition then you can use codes that describe symptoms (e.g. 786.07 *Wheezing*). The V codes can be used for visits, which may not deal with injury or illness (e.g. V20.2 *Routine infant or child health check*).

The ICD-9 code for the main reason for a particular visit should be listed first. Subsequent codes can then follow this code for other conditions or problems that were addressed during the visit.

For example: A patient comes to see you for ear pain and during your examination you discover an acute serous otitis media. During the visit you also discuss the patients benign essential hypertension and recommend lifestyle modifications.

The visit may be coded using the following ICD-9 codes:

381.01 Acute serous otitis media
401.1 Essential hypertension benign

If you are uncertain of a particular diagnosis or need further investigation then you should not use a diagnosis code but a code that describes the presentation.

For example: A 12-year old boy and his mother came to visit you for a chronic cough and periodic wheezing. You are suspicious for asthma but do not have enough information to make the diagnosis yet. You order pulmonary function testing and a chest x-ray to rule-out asthma or other conditions and have the child return the next day.

The visit may be coded using the following codes. The code for asthma should not be used since you are just ruling out (or in) this condition.

786.2 *Cough*
786.07 *Wheezing*

Completing the HCFA1500 Form

The HCFA1500 form (www.cms.gov) is the form used to bill Medicare, Medicaid, and third party insurers. The HCFA1500 form has space for up to four different ICD-9 codes and no more. In some circumstances you may have a patient with more than four conditions that you address during your visit but still you must choose only four codes. You may supply additional documentation and attach it to the HCFA1500 form if you feel the additional information is essential for the claim to be processed. The ICD-9 codes should be listed in order in box 21 of the HCFA1500 filing form (*See Appendix M*).

Each procedure or service that you perform should be represented by an ICD-9 code that substantiates that particular procedure.

CPT® Coding (Services and Procedures)

The American Medical Association has developed the uniform coding system known as CPT coding. All reimbursable provider services have a CPT code and all insurance carriers recognize the CPT codes. The purpose of the CPT code is to provide a recognized language in describing medical, surgical, and diagnostic services that allows for easy communication between providers, patients, and third parties such as the insurance industry. In other words CPT codes describe what was done during the visit. The CPT codes are now on their 4th edition since their inception in 1966 and are revised to some degree annually.

The use of CPT codes allows for an adequate and simplified reporting of services or procedures to Medicare, Medicaid and third parties for reimbursement. The CPT code is a numerical five-digit code. The CPT codes are separated into groups as follows:

99201-99499	Evaluation and Management
00100-01999, 99100-99140	Anesthesiology
10021-69990	Surgery
70010-79999	Radiology
80048-89399	Laboratory
90281-99199, 99500-99569	Medicine

E&M (Evaluation & Management) Codes

The E&M codes are the "bread and butter" codes for nurse practitioners because they are the codes used most often. The E&M codes describe the professional services of evaluating and managing symptoms or disease. In other words, this is the service in which you examine the patient, take a history, and formulate a diagnosis and treatment plan. Although the E&M codes are the most frequently used CPT codes they can be the most difficult to learn. Become familiar with both the 1995 and 1997 versions of the CMS documentation guidelines easily obtained at www.cms.hhs.gov.

Breaking Down the E&M Codes

The E&M codes are separated into several categories such as office visits, hospital visits, consultations, and others.

e.g.

99201-99215 Office or Other Outpatient Services
99221-99239 Hospital Inpatient Services
99421-99275 Consultations

The categories are then divided into subcategories.

e.g.

99211-99215 Established Patient Office or Other
Outpatient Services

The subcategories are then further classified into levels.

e.g.

99214 Detailed Established Patient Office or Other
Outpatient Services

Selecting the correct E&M code

The process of selecting the correct E&M code increases
in difficulty as you further define the code.

Step One. Start first with selecting the location of
service. In most cases this will be in the office or an
outpatient setting (99201-99205).

Step Two. Next determine whether the visit is with a
new patient (not seen by anyone in your group in the
past 3 years) or established patient. The majority of
nurse practitioners patients will fall under the
established patient category 99211-99215 in the office
setting. [No distinction is made between new or
established patient in the emergency department
setting.]

Step Three. The last step is the most complicated. This
involves selecting the level of service that is appropriate
for the visit. There are five different levels of services

that are defined by the degree of complexity of the visit in an outpatient office setting and can simply be defined as limited, basic, expanded, detailed, and comprehensive. The degree of complexity is based on several factors including history, examination, medical decision making, counseling, coordination of care, nature of presenting problem, and time. The history, examination, and medical decision-making are the key features used in selecting a code while the other factors can be considered contributory (the exception to this are visits which consist predominately of counseling).

History

The extent of the history obtained is determined by the provider in relation to the presenting problem for that visit. For example a less extensive history is needed on someone presenting with a finger laceration as opposed to someone presenting with chest pressure. The extent of the history obtained can be defined by four categories:

Problem focused: Consisting of a chief complaint and brief history of present illness.

Expanded problem focused: Consisting of a chief complaint, brief history of present illness, and a problem specific review of systems.

Detailed: Consisting of a chief complaint, an extended history of present illness, a problem specific review of systems with review of a few other systems, pertinent past, social, and/or family history which relate to the problem being addressed.

Comprehensive: Consisting of a chief complaint, extended history of present illness, comprehensive review of systems pertinent to the problem addressed with the addition of the review of all other systems, and a complete past medical, family and social history.

Examination

The extent of the examination is also determined by the provider, based on the presenting problem. The examination can be classified into the same 4 categories:

Problem focused: Consisting of a limited examination of the injured or affected area.

Expanded problem focused: Consisting of a limited examination of the affected area and other related systems or areas.

Detailed: Consisting of an examination of the affected area and extended to other affected areas or related areas or systems.

Comprehensive: Consisting of a general multi-system examination or complete examination of the affected organ system.

The CPT coding guidelines recognize the following as systems or areas to be examined: -Head -Neck –Chest -Abdomen -Genitalia –Back -Extremities –Eyes –Ears, Nose, Throat, Mouth –Cardiovascular –Respiratory –Gastrointestinal –Genitourinary –Musculoskeletal –Skin –Neurologic –Psychiatric –Hematologic, Lymphatic, Immunologic. It is important to keep this in mind during your documentation process.

Time

Time can also be used as a factor in determining the level of E&M code that you use. This can be difficult. The documented time must be the time spent face to face with the provider and should be described in nature (such as coordinating home health care or counseling regarding diet and lifestyle change in relation to hypertension).

Limited >15 minutes, Basic >30 minutes, Expanded >40 minutes, Detailed >60 minutes, Comprehensive >80 minutes

Medical Decision Making

The degree of medical complexity is also divided into four categories: straightforward, low complexity, moderate complexity, and high complexity. Selecting the medical decision making complexity level is based on three factors: the number of diagnoses or management options, the amount or complexity of data to be reviewed by the provider (medical records, diagnostic tests, etc.), and the risk of significant complications or morbidity/mortality. In order to qualify for a given level of decision-making, two of the three elements must be met at the same level or exceeded. For example to meet the criteria for moderate complexity decision making, then at least 2 of the following 3 elements must be met or exceeded: a moderate level of risk, a moderate amount or complexity of data to be reviewed, and multiple diagnosis or management options.

Selecting the appropriate level of E&M code is also based on the categories and subcategories already defined.

For example, in relation to office visits: A new patient office visit will require that all of the key components including history, examination, and medical decision making meet or exceed the requirements to qualify for a particular level of E&M service. Thus, for a detailed E&M level (99204) to be met there must be a comprehensive history, a comprehensive examination, and medical decision making of moderate complexity. However, if the patient was an established patient then only 2 of 3 of the key components must be met. Thus, for a detailed E&M level (99214) two of the three following has to be met; a detailed history, a detailed examination, and moderate complexity decision-making.

Realize that this is the most difficult area of coding to grasp and there is not always agreement on the level of E&M codes. The complexity of decision-making can be somewhat of a subjective measurement since there are not specific measurable criteria for level of risk or complexity of data to be reviewed. Review the clinical examples in *Appendix I* to get a general grasp for what patient visit types fall under the various established office visit E&M levels. A pocket-sized worksheet may be helpful (*Appendix J*) or if you are more techno savvy handheld software applications are available as well (www.handheldmed.com). You should be familiar with your use of the different E & M levels. The majority of primary care providers will have a bell curve look to their E & M patterns with mostly level 3's, a lot of level 2's and 4's and a few level 1's and 5's.

Use of Procedure Codes

Uses of the other CPT codes are easier to select and simply consist of finding the right CPT code to identify the procedure, which was performed. For example, if during a well child exam you gave an IPV immunization you would include the CPT code 90713 (Poliovirus vaccine, inactivated, for subcutaneous use). Once you become familiar with codes you commonly use you can make yourself a pocket card or place them on your "Superbill". A superbill serves as a receipt for your patient and sort of a charge slip for your office. Most offices will have these if they are not yet computerized (*Appendix H*).

Modifiers Mayhem

While there are thousands of CPT codes to use for the reimbursement of services, it's the modifiers that can add the extra detail and reimbursement for a visit. A modifier serves as an addendum to CPT codes and indicates that the service or procedure has been altered in some way. In other words it further defines a service. The CPT code must still accurately define the procedure or service performed, the modifier just says something is different than usual. For example the –25 modifier applies when a significant separately identifiable service is performed by the same provider on the same day of another procedure or service. For instance a patient is in your office for an annual exam and you noticed an unusually shaped lesion, which you remove during the visit. You can bill for the appropriate E & M service and for the lesion removal procedure by attaching the –25 modifier. Without adding the modifier most payers will bundle the two separate services assuming the procedure was part of the exam and thus resulting in a lower reimbursement. Other examples include when a service or procedure is performed more than once during the visit (modifier –59) or when two different surgeons are performing two distinct parts of the same surgery on a patient the same day (modifier –62).

Unlisted Procedures or Services

When a procedure or service is performed that does not have a CPT listing then there are a few code numbers that can be used to bill for the procedure/service. The code should then be followed by an explanation of what was done. The majority and maybe all of the services or procedures you provide will have their own number. If there is no code then look for an unlisted code located in the section where you would find the procedure or service if there was a code. One example is code 90799 described as *Unlisted therapeutic, prophylactic or diagnostic injection.*

Completing the HCFA1500 Form

CPT codes are listed in section 24 of the HCFA1500 form. The diagnosis (ICD-9) code, which relates to the procedure (CPT) code should be linked by placing the ranked number of the ICD-9 (1,2,3,4) in the box entitled "diagnosis code" located next to the CPT code box. Section 24 contains room for 6 separate CPT codes.

HCFA Common Procedure Coding System

HCPCS or the Common Procedure Coding System was added in 1983 by HCFA, which we now call CMS. The purpose of HCPCS was to standardize codes for Medicare processing that are not located in the CPT manual. Technically the CPT codes fall under the heading of the HCPCS coding system labeled *Level 1* but it is simpler to think of them separately. The HCPCS coding system is divided into three levels including the CPT codes as level 1, the level II codes pertaining mostly to supplies, materials, and injections, and the level III codes which allow the local Medicare carriers to identify services that are particular to a certain area. Note that not all of HCPCS codes are covered by Medicare. The HCPCS level II codes are organized in a similar fashion as the CPT codes and consist of a 5-digit alphanumeric code including a letter followed by 4 numbers. The following is a listing of the various sections in the HCPCS level II coding publications.

A0000-A0999 Transportation services
A2000-A2999 Chiropractic Services
A4000-A4999 Medical and Surgical Supplies
A9000-A9999 Miscellaneous and Experimental
B4000-B9999 Enteral and Parenteral Therapy
C0000-C9999 Temporary Hospital Outpatient
D0000-D9999 Dental Procedures
E0000-E9999 Durable Medical Equipment

G0000-G9999 Procedure/Services Temporary
H5000-H5999 Rehabilitative Services
J0000-J8999 Drugs Administered other than Oral Route
J9000-J9999 Chemotherapy Drugs
K0000-K9999 Temporary Codes for Durable Medical
Equipment Regional Carriers
L0000-L4999 Orthotic Procedures
L5000-L9999 Prosthetic Procedures
M0000-M9999 Medical Services
P0000-P9999 Pathology and Laboratory
Q0000-Q0099 Temporary Codes
R0000-R5999 Diagnostic Radiology Services
S0000-S9999 Private Payer Codes
V0000-V2999 Vision Services
V5000-V5999 Hearing Services

The Most Important Lessons in Coding

Documentation

The single most important lesson about billing and
coding is to adequately document what it is you do.
Nurses are trained from the start about the importance
of accurate medical documentation and it can help us
both financially and legally now in the nurse
practitioner profession. Documentation is the only
evidence that payers have to show what was done and
whether what was done is supported by medical
necessity. Correct billing documentation is just as
important as traditional medical documentation when it
comes to medico legal issues.

Do Not Up-Code

J.R. Ewing from the well-acclaimed show "Dallas" once
stated that "Once you loose your integrity the rest
comes easy". So, maintain your integrity.

Up-coding is the term used for billing at a higher level of service than that performed or billing for services never done. Not only is this plain un-ethical it is illegal. Nurse practitioner providers will likely receive even more scrutiny than their physician counterparts during an audit. Never, ever, ever up-code. The most frequent area where up-coding is found to occur is with the E&M codes. Always make sure your documentation and the care you provide supports the level of E&M code selected.

Do Not Down-Code

Down-Coding is the term used for billing for a lower level of service than that provided. Most nurse practitioners are more apt to down-code for the fear that they may accidentally up-code. Billing for a lower level of service can be as drastic as the above by decreasing practice income and thus not justifying your role. If the visit meets the guidelines of a certain level and this is well documented then the visit should be billed at that level. Many practices have resorted to just billing all their visits at a certain level thus minimizing insurance carrier scrutiny, but this is not good practice. First, billing all visits at the same level often triggers an audit. Second, billing at one level will not guarantee insurance carrier automatic payment.

Do Not Ignore the Subject of Coding

You may feel confident that you have qualified coders who work for you but don't use this as an excuse not to learn the coding process. The provider (that's you) is the responsible party for assuring the coding is done correctly. Ignorance is not an appropriate excuse when fraud occurs. Your knowledge of coding and billing issues will increase your worth to the practice. Very few physicians enjoy this aspect of practicing medicine as well.

Always Be As Specific As Possible

Code to the highest level of specificity possible with ICD-9 codes and CPT codes.

Link Your Codes

Be sure to link tests/procedures ordered or performed to an appropriate ICD-9 code. This will help justify the reason for the test/procedure (CPT code).

Use All the Resources Available

Computerized coding and documentation systems will pay for themselves and allow you to be more productive and spend more time with your patients. Don't be afraid to consult your coding manuals especially with diagnoses and codes less familiar to you.

Perform Ongoing Internal Audits

Internal audits can catch potential problems. If performed prior to billing, audits may save you from generating false claims and may increase your revenue by catching undercoding.

Business Essentials for Nurse Practitioners
116

Chapter 9

Building a Solo Practice

"Not only believe in miracles but rely on them."

The African Impala

The African Impala is a wonderful deer like animal
residing in Southern Africa. Although the Impala does
not look that much different from a deer, other than its
peculiar antlers, it has tremendous capabilities. In a
single leap the Impala can jump over 8 feet high and 30
feet long. Despite this great leaping ability, however, the
Impala can be easily contained in a zoo environment.
The Impala is often contained with nothing more than a
three-foot high fencing. The zookeepers know the
Impala can easily jump over this fencing but it chooses
not to. Why is it that the Impala chooses not to leap
over the fencing? Because the Impala must be able to
see where it will land before it leaps. The Impala lacks
faith and is unwilling to take the risk of leaping where it
is not sure where it will end up landing. The Impala
would never choose to be in solo practice because it
lacks the entrepreneurial quality of risk taking.
Webster's Dictionary defines an entrepreneur as "one
who organizes, manages, and assumes risk of a business
or enterprise".

Building a solo practice is not an easy task for the
physician let alone the NP. Multiple barriers exist for
the clinician initiating such an endeavor. Foremost,
nurse practitioners have yet to gain the respect they
deserve as independent providers, which often results in
inadequate reimbursement by insurance providers and
public ignorance of what we do. Additionally, over half
of all new businesses in the United States fail in the first
year and a half and of those who do survive the first
year, fail within the next five years.

This chapter is not only written for the nurse
practitioner considering starting an independent
practice but for those who work as employees as well.
Having a knowledge of the process of initiating and
maintaining a business will give you respect for all that

is involved. There are currently well under 2% of NP's who actually own their own practice.

Are *You* Ready to Start Your Own Practice

Whether you are prepared to start your own business will likely rely on several key issues including your financial situation, personal life situation and the degree of determination and motivation you have. Starting an independent practice is certainly not for everyone and you must really be willing to take a significant degree of risk. Weighing the pros and cons of working independently versus working as an employee is a process we all go through at least in our heads. Some may come to a conclusion with minimal thought when faced with the uncertainty of how well a private practice may do. Others may want to take more time to think and even write down the strengths and weakness of independent practice to determine if they are ready to take the plunge. Consider the sacrifices you may have to make as a small business owner, the risks involved with starting a new business venture, the support system you have in place, and the special skills you have that may set you apart from the other providers in your area. A helpful task during your decision process may be to write down the pros and cons of independent practice as you see them against each other.

Business Essentials for Nurse Practitioners

PROS	Independent Practice	CONS
- Independence		- Security
- Flexibility		- Administrative Demands
- Chance for Higher Income		- Benefits

Business Formations

Choosing a business form

Care should be taken when deciding which corporate form to utilize while operating your business venture. Many experts recommend consultation with a lawyer or certified public accountant to assist with this decision. Business forms are usually categorized as either informal or formal with the differentiation often being that formal associations require the filing of organizational documents with the Secretary of State. Most successful practices end up as a corporation but this does not mean you have to start as one. Your first decision on a business formation does not have to be your last one. Many small businesses start as sole proprietors then change to a formal business entity once the business has been established.

Informal Associations

Sole Proprietorship: One person who conducts business for profit. The sole owner assumes complete responsibility for all liabilities and debts of the business. The income of the business is reported as part of the owner's personal income.

General Partnership: Two or more individuals as co-owners of a for-profit business. Partnerships should operate under a written partnership agreement to avoid future problems. All partners are responsible for the liabilities and debts of the partnership. Partnerships enjoy single taxation like sole proprietorship. Income is reported as part of each partner's personal income.

Formal Associations

Limited Liability Partnership (LLP): A general partnership, which elects to operate as an LLP. To operate as an LLP, a registration must be filed with the Secretary of State. Unlike a general partnership described above, the partners in an LLP enjoy protection from many of the partnership's debts and liabilities. The income of an LLP is taxed in the same manner as a general partnership.

Limited Partnership: A partnership with at least one general partner and one limited partner. A limited partner's liability is limited to the amount invested, while the general partner(s) assumes all the liabilities and debts of the partnership. The income is taxed in the same manner as a general partnership.

Corporation: A legal entity, which is created by filing articles of incorporation. The Corporation itself, assumes all liabilities and debts of the Corporation. A Corporation is owned by shareholders. A shareholder enjoys protection from the corporation's debts and liabilities. There is an option of having just one shareholder. Income is taxed twice, first at the corporate level and then the employee level when a wage is paid or at the shareholder level when distributed as a dividend.

S-Corporation: After filing articles of incorporation, a Corporation may seek to obtain S Corporation status, for federal income tax purposes. The income of an S Corporation is taxed only once: at the employee or shareholder level. To qualify, the corporation may not have more than 75 shareholders and must meet other certain Internal Revenue Service criteria. The Corporation must submit IRS form #2553 to the IRS. An S Corporation is considered a corporation in all other aspects and is subject to no additional or special filing requirements with the Secretary of State.

Nonprofit Corporation: A corporation whose purpose is to engage in activities, which do not provide financial profit to the benefit of its members. Such corporations must obtain nonprofit or tax exempt status from the IRS and State Department of Revenue, to be free from certain tax burdens.

Limited Liability Company (LLC): An LLC is a formal association, which combines the advantage of a corporation's limited liability and the flexibility and single taxation of a general partnership. An LLC has members, rather than shareholders. A member enjoys protections from the liabilities and debts of the LLC. Although not required by law, an LLC should operate under an Operating Agreement much like a Partnership Agreement. If the LLC qualifies under IRS guidelines, it may be taxed only once, like a partnership, at the employee or member level while not having the same restrictions as an S-Corporation.

Surveying the Market

The demand for your services must be present if your business is going to succeed. Determining whether there is a demand for your services should be done before your decision to go into independent practice. Before beginning an analysis of your target market you should have already developed an idea for your intended services. That is, what is it that you intend to provide or sell. You may decide to open a practice focused on your training such as family practice, women's health, pediatrics, or geriatrics. You may also decide to specialize in the care of certain disease entities such as diabetes, obesity, or fibromyalgia. The basis for your decision should not only reflect your interests but also the market where you intend to practice.

In order for your business to survive in the market area you wish to establish your practice the area must be able to support another practice or be inadequately supported by the existing practices. A survey of your potential market can be done in several different fashions and should not rely on only one.

Window Survey

A window survey is just as it sounds, surveying a particular area through the window of your car. Grab your local phone book and a map of the area you wish to serve. Next drive around your potential market area surveying the established practices and marking them on your map. When you are finished visiting all the existing practices then visit the areas that are absent of an existing practice and evaluate whether there is a need for the practice you wish to establish.

Census data reviews

Your local librarian can assist you with reviewing the census of zip codes in your area. This information can be very helpful together with your window survey in determining heavily populated areas where no current practices are located.

Develop a Strategic Plan

Establish in your mind where you want your business to be. Once you have determined that an independent practice has potential and are committed to realizing your dream then your first step should be to start planning.

Writing a "Business Plan"

Successful businesses begin with the development of a comprehensive business plan. A business plan serves multiple purposes and is a must for every business. Foremost, the business plan serves to establish the direction you take during start up and will make you address several key areas of business development you may otherwise avoid addressing. A good business plan is also essential in acquiring loans and relaying your goals to the accountants, lawyers, and anyone else you will work with.

The process of writing your business plan may involve the assistance of an accountant or lawyer but the first draft should be done by yourself. Only you know how you want your business to look and function. The actual writing of the plan can be directed by reading one of several books on the subject or with the use of business plan writing software (Microsoft Small Office Tools®). A sample plan is located in *Appendix F.*

Business Basics

Selecting a Name for Your Business

Law requires that the name of a Corporation, L.P., L.L.C. and an L.L.P. must be distinguishable from the names of other businesses of the same type. Search the web site or call your state's Secretary of State office for information on name checks or applications to reserve names. You may also want to seek consultation with an attorney who specializing in copyright law. The name of your practice should distinguish you in some way from other practices and at the same time tell the potential customer what it is you do. Common errors in developing a name include making the name to long or complicated. Keep your name short and easy for the consumer to understand. Run your name by several lay people as well as medical professionals before you make your decision. Your name will be hard to change once you have begun to practice and establish your business.

Continuing Responsibilities

After its initial organization, formal businesses must continue to meet certain statutory requirements. Requirements will vary by state and you should seek direction from a good CPA (certified public accountant) who you will likely need at some point in the process of starting a new business. You might as well start at the beginning stages.

Marketing

Marketing in today's business world is not an option even among professional corporations. Many business plans include a section for marketing but this is one area, which deserves a separate plan and focused attention. An important aspect for the independent nurse practitioner is establishing a niche or unique focus that will grab the attention of your potential clients. Use this unique aspect of your practice in developing a sales pitch. A sales pitch says "why you" in one brief statement. An example of a sales pitch for the business described in the sample business plan is "Caring for You with the Balance of Alternative and Traditional Medicine".

Accounting

A good accountant is a must but the majority of the checks and balances will likely be performed by you or your business manager (if you have one). Again you can and should make use of available computer programs. A good accounting program is well worth the small investment and makes the process of "keeping the books" simple *(QuickBooks Pro®, Simply Accounting®)*. All good accountants are familiar with these programs and it will make their job easier as well when it comes to tax time.

Collaborative Agreements/Hiring Professional Services of a Physician

Most states require nurse practitioners collaborate with a physician to practice. Independent nurse practitioners will then have to establish a relationship with a physician and likely pay them for their services. For instance it may be required that a physician review at least 5% of your records where treatment was prescribed. You can set up a contract where you pay the physician for each chart reviewed or pay them a monthly fee for reviewing your charts.

Research the current laws and practice acts in your state and seek legal counsel. It is important to find a lawyer who is knowledgeable with nurse practitioner practice.

Licenses

Your business will likely need to apply for an Employer Identification Number (EIN), which serves to identify you as an employer. Many banks require this number to open a business account and often times businesses you work with will use this number to establish accounts with your business. The EIN is used for tax purposes most importantly. Additional licenses you may need to set up include:

Clinical Laboratory Improvement Amendment (CLIA) Certificate of Registration. If you will be performing any sort of laboratory work within your office setting (including CLIA waved testing) you will need to register with CLIA. There are different levels of registration dependent upon the complexity of testing you plan to do within your practice. Information can be obtained off of CLIA's web site (www.fda.gov/cdrh/clia).

Biohazard Waste Generator Permit. You will need to check with your state office as to whether this is required. You will most definitely need to establish a relationship with a hazardous waste company to pick up and dispose of the hazardous waste that is generated (unless the medical office you lease already has this in place for you).

Federal, State, and local licenses

Check with your local Chamber of Commerce with regard to which licenses may be required for you to be open for business in your practice location.

Essential Forms

HCFA 1500, Patient intake, Initial H/P, Prescription pads, Telephone call forms, Consent forms, Visit forms, Superbills, Patient instruction hand outs.

Essential Reference Books

Physicians Desk Reference, CPT, ICD-9, Diagnostic Reference, Primary Care Reference, Emergency Care Reference

Billing for Services

There are several ways to set up billing for your services. You will have to make the decision of whether to set up relationships with third party payers in order to receive payment from HMO's, PPO's, Medicare, Medicaid and other health insurance organizations. It is always a good idea to accept private pay patients, which gives you payment at the time of services (that is unless you want to set up payment plans with patients).

Accepting Private Pay

Credit Card Acceptance

Credit cards increase sales and increase the size of the sale while it cuts down on collection problems. People have become accustomed to using credit cards for payment, which makes it essential for you to accept them. In order to accept payment via credit cards you will have to set up a Merchant Account with a bank. Preferably you can do this at your own bank but you

may need to research a few others to compare costs.
The majority of banks charge a set up fee and then a
monthly fee that may correlate with the amount of
transactions you make. The bank will set you up with a
scanner which either works through a phone line or
through a personal computer. The Merchant Payment
Scanner or Software allows you to run credit cards
through to verify validity of the card and then
transmission of funds to your account. You will have to
decide which credit cards to accept such as VISA®,
MasterCard®, American Express®, and Discover®, which
are listed in order of most widely used. Agreeing to
accept payment from these credit cards means that you
agree to accept the discount associated with the
particular cards. The discounts range from 3-7% of each
transaction dependent upon the amount of the sale,
your monthly volume and the particular card. The
upside is that your account is credited immediately.
Accepting credit cards will increase your cash flow and
may decrease your need for expensive short-term loans
as you start your practice.

Accepting Personal Checks and Cash

Accepting personal checks also gives you payment
quickly but comes with a little risk (the risk of a
returned check). Generally speaking medical offices
receive less returned checks than the majority of
businesses and it is probably worth the small risk.
Accepting cash is a given in any business but be sure
the transaction is recorded accurately. All patients
should be provided with a "superbill" which lists the
diagnoses, the procedures and services rendered, the
amount paid, and often times when their next
appointment is due. A "superbill" can be hand generated
(*Appendix H*) or computer generated and can serve as a
receipt for the patient.

Accepting Third-Party Payment

The decision to accept third-party reimbursement may be determined by the third party payer. Some NP's in private practice try to just stay away from the "red tape" of third-party reimbursement and only accept payment at time of service. In order to build a fair sized practice, however, it may be a good idea to at least investigate third-party contracts. Medicare and Medicaid very rarely turn down NP providers so start with them.

Establishing Your Rates

An independent nurse practitioner will likely have to be fairly competitive with regard to their fee schedule. Legally, medical offices should not discuss their fee schedules with other practices. You will probably have an idea of what the other providers in your area are charging by the rates you were charged as a patient or by your previous experience. You can really choose to set your prices how you see fit and you can adjust your fee schedule up and down just so long as you charge everyone the same fees. Medicare lists what they pay for certain CPT codes on their website which can certainly be a starting point. Many practices base their rates by multiplying Medicare allowable by a certain percentage such as 125%-200%.

Establishing Your Office Setting

Geographic Location

Geographic considerations are frequently influenced by such factors as family, recreational areas, housing availability, cost of living, and the results of your market survey. Once you have found the general area, which you would like to practice, the search begins to find an office setting.

Office Space

Options on obtaining office space include buying, leasing, or sharing office space. Buying space will not likely be an option for a start-up business unless you have a substantial amount of investment money to start your practice with. Sharing office space can be a good idea so long as the practice you share space with is not a competing business. Sharing a space may allow you to begin part-time until you establish patients and are able to afford leasing a full-time office. The advantages of leasing include having an identified office of your own and the ability to construct or renovate it the way that works best for your practice. The most important aspects of choosing an office will be the location, costs, and the functionality and current condition of the facility. Consider having a lawyer review any lease or agreement you are considering.

Office Supplies

There are multiple equipment and supply needs for a medical practice. The majority of these materials will be needed before you open your practice doors. Many of your equipment and supply needs can be purchased as used or donated by yourself or others. Essentials will include at least one personal computer, several phones and phone lines, a fax machine, furnishings and medical supplies.

Financing

Determining Start-Up Costs

Starting a new practice involves a substantial amount of start up money. You may or may not have enough money of your own to get your practice started. Generally speaking, the costs associated with starting an independent practice will be more than you expect. Before seeking funding for your new business you should have some idea of the initial start-up costs and average monthly expenses. It is very difficult to estimate or know how much will be needed to fund your new business but an effort should be made to look at all the expenses that your are aware of. The form in *Appendix E* can be used to help remember many of the operating expenses of a medical practice but will probably not cover all of them.

Obtaining Start-Up Funding

Many new businesses begin with funds from their own bank account but this is not always possible unless you have been planning and saving for some time. Small loans can be obtained from local or international banks as well as through the Small Business Administration (www.sba.gov). Research your funding options before you sign the papers on a large loan with a large annual percentage rate and seek the consultation of your accountant.

Keys Step toward Success

Provide quality care

To become a successful solo practitioner, the most important practice is to provide high-quality patient care. Keep up to date in your field by attending conferences and reviewing appropriate journals on an ongoing basis.

Be a patient advocate

The deliverance of superior care that is proven through outcomes requires being an outspoken patient advocate. Your ongoing journal reading will lead to treatment modalities that you would not have thought of before which will end up benefiting many of your patients.

Be available and accessible

Availability and accessibility are reliable practice builders that will also improve the care you provide. Be available to see new patients within 24 hours. Patients should know they can reach you in 20-30 minutes at all times so buy a pager. You can always send emergency situations to the emergency room but patients like talking to their own provider first if that option is available to them.

Provide personalized care

Personalized care is always a top priority. Patients appreciate that you know them personally. On the same hand they usually connect with you better if they know you personally. A good start is by including a picture of yourself on a marketing resume and including your hobbies or interests allowing them to connect with you on a more personal level. Conversing with them about events in your own life reminds patients that you are human. Discuss something personal during every visit showing your interest in him or her as a whole person. Don't forget to truly listen to your patients. Two minutes of active listening will create a better relationship with your patients than ½ an hour spent of you talking.

Provide cost-effective care

As a sole practitioner you can provide better continuity of care with increased cost effectiveness.

Provide "outrageously great service"

Truly great service is from the heart. Be aware of and ask about service breakdowns in your office. When you discover a problem then fix it by looking at the patient's perspective first and foremost.

Have a sense of humor

A good sense of humor and a positive attitude will go a long way. Don't forget to allow your staff to have an appropriate amount of freedom to have fun at work as well.

Create a Unique "Niche"

If you are the only person in the city specializing in fibromyalgia then make it well known.

Management Mastery

Learning effective management skills is not an easy process and one that may not be possible to learn without experience. Including management techniques in this book would add another 100 pages but here are a few key important ingredients.

Hire the right people and treat them well. Your employees will become your business' greatest asset if you train them and treat them right.

Pay attention to the numbers and details. Do not rely on others to make sure all the checks and balances are correct and in order. As a business owner this is your responsibility.

The more attention you pay to a behavior the more it will by repeated. Accentuate the positive.

Make informed decisions based on both quality and cost.

Market to grow. You must market intensely as you start your business and never stop marketing as it grows. Marketing works, that's why we do not have to pay for local television and radio.

Dress in business attire. Dress like a professional to be respected as a professional.

Ask your happy patients for their referrals. Never underestimate the power of a patient referral. People usually trust their friends over an article, ad, or even a respected journal article.

Catch employees doing things right instead of naturally catching them doing wrong.

Health plan enrollment. To gain access to patients, many practitioners choose to enroll in all available plans. On the same note make sure you read and understand every detail of a contract.

Chapter 10

Corporate Compliance/Malpractice

There is never a situation where you should say "I'm new at this".

Corporate Compliance

The federal crackdown on Medicare fraud and abuse has invoked fear of an audit for many practitioners and physicians. The sample compliance program for small practices released last year by the Officer of Inspector General (OIG) lists seven key components of a compliance program (www.hhs.gov.progorg/oig). The OIG recognizes that the scope and size of an organization may limit its resources for establishing and maintaining a compliance program. The OIG still expects smaller practices to make some effort to establish a compliance plan. You should not assume that the size of your practice will protect you from investigation. The seven key components are meant to be recommendations and practices are not required to take the advice. The components include:

• Conducting internal monitoring and auditing.

• Implementing compliance and practice standards.

• Designating a compliance officer or contact.

• Conducting appropriate training and education.

• Responding appropriately to detected offenses and developing corrective action.

• Developing open lines of communication.

• Enforcing disciplinary standards through well-publicized guidelines.

Chart Auditing

Practices that audit frequently may actually realize an economic benefit. Remember that audits catch under-billing just as frequently as over-billing especially among nurse practitioners. There are other benefits to performing audits such as discovering information you did not see during the visit, catching missed follow up appointments or follow up on lab work and opportunities to make improvements in documentation forms etc. The OIG gives no recommendation on the frequency or amount of chart auditing that should be performed. A good rule of thumb is to perform audits on 10-20 charts quarterly for each provider in your practice. The charts should not be "cherry picked" but chosen in some random fashion. Audits can be performed by in-house personnel or by a hired agency. An outside agency may be more expensive but you wont have to worry about training staff or staff being afraid to contradict their providers.

What are you looking for during an audit?

-Coding and Billing. Services are coded and billed correctly with appropriate modifiers.

-Documentation is completed correctly. Documents are legible and include the reason for visit, relevant history, the exam, testing, diagnosis, plan of care, date, provider identification, rational for testing, etc.

-The services performed are reasonable and necessary. (e.g. there is a proper ICD-9 to go along with the procedures performed.)

-Improper self-referrals or kickbacks.

Developing Standards

A practice should initiate a corporate compliance program starting with practice standards and procedures in written form. To start the standards should determine how records will be selected for audit, how many records will be audited, procedures to take when errors are found, and the performance of staff training. Included in the standards may be auditing tools (*Appendix K*) and procedures for retaining, creating and destruction of records. Additionally, the standards should put in writing the provider's commitment to compliance with all state and federal statutes, rules, and regulations. The standards should be distributed to all employees. A statement certifying the employee has received, read, understood, and has agreed to the standards should be signed by each employee and placed in their employee record.

Designate a Compliance Officer

A compliance officer can consist of one person responsible for the whole program or several people responsible for different aspects of the program. An non-staff member can be designated as the practices compliance officer but they have to be familiar with the routines and "inner workings" or functions of your practice. The duties of the compliance officer include but are not "limited to":

-Overseeing periodic audits.

-Revising the compliance program when needed.

-Developing or organizing staff training in relation to corporate compliance.

-Investigating reports of improper business practices.

-Taking corrective action when errors or improper practices have occurred.

Conducting Appropriate Training and Education

Training and education with regard to corporate compliance should be reoccurring according to the OIG (such as annually). Training can be performed in-house by the compliance officer or by outside sources.

Educational topics should include at least the following:

-Proper documentation for services rendered.

-Applicable sanctions and regulations.

-The operation and importance of the compliance program along with its benefits.

-Legal sanctions for submitting deliberately false or inaccurate billings.

-Information discovered during a random internal audit.

Responding to Detected Violations

The corporate compliance standards should in detail explain the process of responding to discovered violations. The process should include three basic steps: Step one involves the investigation of a potential problem to be sure it truly exists. Step two is correcting the problem identified immediately. The last step is determining whether self-disclosure should occur and whether you contact a lawyer.

In summary, remember that it is the provider who is ultimately responsible and that a good compliance program is a good business decision. A good compliance program will protect you more than hurt you. Encourage employees to notify the compliance officer of potential problems. Be sure employees are aware that their anonymity will be kept as best possible and no retribution will occur for truthful information. Compliance efforts should be coordinated with third party billing services if possible to keep communication open and easy.

Medicare and Insurance Audits

In 1996, a massive government audit of Medicare payments revealed over $24 billion in incorrect payments. As a result of this audit Medicare developed a mechanism, whereby claims are run through a "filtering system" or "audit system" before payment occurs. This filtering system has been successful enough that insurance carriers are beginning to do the same. The internal audit system builds a database or "profile" of each provider which tracks billing code utilization. The program then can identify statistical outliers who are flagged for more stringent audit. Circumstances often raising red flags include the repetitive billing of the same codes, a high percentage of claims for one procedure, an unusual procedure from your norm, and a high number of claims or patients coming from one provider. Other leads that may lead to an audit include problems reported by patients, another provider, employees or even professional whistleblowers.

HIPAA Compliance

The latest regulatory challenge facing providers is the Health Insurance Portability and Accountability Act (HIPAA). HIPAA was enacted by Congress in 1996 when the healthcare industry could unsuccessfully agree to standardization. HIPAA sets forth requirements for the Department of Health and Human Services (DHHS) to coordinate standard transactions and codes for the health care industry. Transactions refer mostly to claims and inquiries while codes refer to the common ICD-9 and CPT billing codes you should now be familiar with.

Realizing that electronic transactions are becoming commonplace, Congress also initiated new privacy provisions as well. The privacy provisions not only cover billing transactions but all healthcare information. Healthcare providers have 2 years to comply with the Privacy Rule finalized in April of 2001. The Privacy Rule consists of four major components:

1). Consent and authorization

All patients should sign a consent form allowing anyone involved in healthcare operations access to patient information. An additional form must be signed by the patient if medical information is provided for reasons other than the provision of health care services (such as research).

2). Minimum necessary uses and disclosures

This portion of the Privacy Rule states that persons only have access to or access information that is vital to their performance in their health care role. Large organizations should make information inaccessible if possible to those persons who do not need the information. Smaller organizations will likely just be required to initiate policies stating that employees will only access information that is vital to their function instead of initiating costly processes, which actually limit their access.

3). Patient Rights

Patients have the right to access a copy of their record and should not be charged fees except those for copying. Patients may also request to add an amendment to their record. Providers may refuse this request but will have to follow an extra set of measures. The provider's office must also keep track of all authorized disclosures of the medical record that is available to the patient.

4). Administrative changes

All practices must identify a staff member as a "privacy officer". This could be your "compliance officer" or office manager. All practices must also draft a policy that describes how patient information is handled. Staff must be trained on these issues via policy review or via seminars or training programs. Medical records must be protected in some manner.

Guidelines have been written by the DHHS for providers to follow. The guidelines frequently state that reasonable changes be made giving the small practice time to comply and realizing limitations of a small practice. HIPAA has also required the DHHS to initiate a Security Rule, however, this has yet to be presented in final form at the time of this writing. The requirements of the Security Rule will likely address electronic information security and backup. Numerous changes are likely to occur as HIPAA evolves and it will be important to stay abreast of the requirements (www.cms.gov/hipaa/).

Malpractice Issues

The topic of malpractice and professional liability is one that most NP's would rather avoid reading about. Fortunately, however, the number of lawsuits filed against NP's has historically been limited when compared to physicians. An estimated one NP for every one hundred MD's is sued for malpractice. The explanation for this may be related to several conditions including a smaller number of practicing NP's in relation to practicing physicians, the acuity of patients seen by NP's, underreporting of such lawsuits to the National Practitioner Data Bank (NPDB), and the known patient satisfaction with NP care. The majority (60%) of claims against physicians also arise from hospital care where NP practice is often limited. The majority of lawsuits dealing with NP's are due to negligence. Negligence is the failure to act as a reasonable person or practitioner in a certain circumstance.

For an actual malpractice lawsuit to be valid four particular elements must occur (Table 1). The first element is the duty to provide care to the person must have been established. In other words a patient-practitioner relationship must have been established. The second element is the breach of duty or failure to provide the standard of care. This can occur either by doing something you should not have or not doing something you should have for the patient. Injury to the patient must also occur and this represents the third needed element. The incurred injury usually will have to consist of a physical injury since psychological damages are difficult to prove. Lastly, the injury to the patient must have been directly caused by the breach of duty by the practitioner.

Table 1. Medical Malpractice Elements

Provider/Patient Relationship

Breach of Standard of Care

Injury to patient

Injury caused by Breach of Care

95% of malpractice cases are settled for a "reasonable" amount out of court. Remember plaintiff attorneys are usually only paid upon winning a case (20-40%) and therefore are not likely to take a case unless they feel they can win. Defense attorneys are generally paid by the hour. Your best prophylaxis against the filing of a malpractice case against you includes 4 important actions:

Establish a good rapport with your patients. A patient is less likely to file a suit against you if they trust you and feel as though you care about them.

Remain competent at what you do. Be knowledgeable of the standard of care for the conditions you treat (such as by following national guidelines). If something falls out of your realm of knowledge then refer appropriately.

Document accurately and comprehensively. The old nursing phrase of "If it is not documented it was not done" still holds true in the NP profession.

Take a course in risk management. Risk management is a set of techniques or behaviors to reduce your risk of being sued. In essence risk management courses teach you why patients become plaintiffs. (www.GEMedicalProtective.com)

Table 2: Most Common Allegations and Risk Management Strategies

Allegation: Failure to diagnose cancer
Risk Mgt.: Offer and document routine cancer screenings

Allegation: Failure to diagnose fracture
Risk Mgt.: Have radiologists review radiographs

Allegation: Improper treatment related to medication side effect, errors in dosing or incorrect selection
Risk Mgt.: Have collaborating physician review and sign off on high-risk drug use such as corticosteroids, warfarin, chemotherapy agents etc.

Allegation: Post-op complication such as bleeding and infection
Risk Mgt.: Include the potential problems during pre-op or pre-procedure discussions

Court/Deposition Preparation

Preparing for a court hearing or deposition can be one of the most dreaded tasks for anyone. Adequately preparing for such a daunting event, however, can put you at greater ease. The first step you take should consist of educating yourself on the course of events and standards of care. Review the patients chart first by yourself and then with your lawyer in an attempt to recollect the events that occurred. A precisely documented visit record will certainly make this easier. Review the standard of care for the condition or symptoms you treated at the time of the visit as well. Recommend experts or documents to your lawyer that support your decisions and to improve your credibility. Next, discuss your case honestly and openly with your lawyer so they can greater assist you. It is generally recommended that you refrain from talking to friends, family, co-workers, and the patient or his/her lawyers.

Once the proceedings begin it is important to maintain a calm and professional demeanor at all times. A professional appearance and mannerism is also important and will greatly affect your credibility during the proceedings, so pay attention to detail. Plaintiff attorneys really know how to put on the pressure and will work to use your words against you, so go slow when answering questions. Do not hesitate to ask the lawyers to rephrase a question or even ask for a short break during a deposition.

Professional Liability Insurance

Nurse practitioners claims have been low and coverage can be found at reasonably low rates in comparison to physicians (www.gemedicalprotective.com, www.nso.com, www.cmfgroup.com). However, the last few years has seen a significant rise in premiums for physicians and to some degree NP's. The rise in premiums has actually forced some physicians out of practice or into early retirement (especially among surgical or obstetrical specialties). Many insurers adjust rates upward for NP's with prescriptive authority or practicing within a specialty setting. While searching for an insurance carrier be familiar with whether the plan is an "occurrence" versus a "claims made" policy (occurrence is usually best), how much coverage you have per claim and aggregate ($1 million/$6 million), and whether you have a say when it comes to settlement. Don't be afraid to ask questions and talk to several companies or representatives.

Types of Liability Policies

All liability policies are not the same. NP's should carefully review their policies annually. There are two main types of policies: occurrence and claims made. An occurrence policy covers NP's for claims arising from medical incidents occurring between the policy inception date and expiration date. So long as the claim pertains to an incident that occurred during the policy period it is covered under the policy. A claims made policy, however, only cover claims that arise from a medical incident during the policy period and also filed during the same period of time. It is thus very important to renew claims made policies with a retroactive date if this is the type of policy you choose. "Tail" insurance may also be purchased to cover retroactive time periods if you choose to cancel a claims made policy.

There is no perfect way to determine how much liability insurance coverage to purchase. Some experts feel if you choose to carry an amount of coverage higher than needed you may actually increase the likelihood that you will be sued (Deep pocket theory). Plaintiff attorneys can obtain the amount of insurance coverage you have to determine whether you are an attractive target for a claim. On the other hand, you want to be sure you have plenty of coverage to protect yourself adequately. Your decision may be based on the area of the country you practice in, the amount of liability exposure you have, and the cost of the policy. Insurance companies often place physicians into premium or liability categories and sometimes do the same for NP's.

Table 2: Liability Class Starting with Highest

Obstetrics
Surgery
Emergency Medicine
Anesthesiology
Cardiology
Internal Medicine
Pediatrics
Occupational Health
Psychiatry

Controlling Liability Premiums

The biggest factor on the medical malpractice insurance industry is obviously the number of lawsuits filed and the amounts actually paid to resolve these claims. The recent wave in large dollar judgments has found many companies with inadequate money reserves leaving them unable to pay off settlements. Several large insurance companies have actually removed themselves from the market. Insurers utilize several assessment tools to determine premium rates in addition to lawsuits filed and amounts paid. One such tool is the review of closed claims where insurers review closed cases to identify allegations per specialty, suits filed with respect to geographic location, amounts paid, and losses related to particular procedures performed. Premium rates thus have little to do with your skills and knowledge as a provider but more to do with the climate of liability within your specialty and geographic location.

The current "hardened" insurance market may actually open up discussion with regard to tort reform. Several states have had success in passing tort reform that essentially places caps on damages. Without limits, the insurance industry becomes unable to cover its obligations, which then results in unreasonable premium to providers. A second solution often discussed involves limiting "contingency fees" paid to plaintiffs' attorneys. Plaintiff attorneys often earn 40-50 percent of a plaintiff's indemnity payment which does very little to support the inured party. The large payout to plaintiff attorneys increases the number of attorneys specializing in this area, which in the end results in more cases. At the time of finishing this book President Bush endorsed a House bill (HR 4600) known as the Help Efficient, Accessible, Low Cost, Timely Health Care (HEALTH) Act. The purpose of the Amendment is to cap the noneconomic damages (pain and suffering) at $250,000. Punitive damages would be limited to the greater of two times the amount of economic damages or $250,000.

Chapter 11

Justifying and Promoting the Nurse Practitioner Profession

"Learn from the mistakes of others. There is not enough time to make them all yourself."

Nurse practitioners have been in existence now for more than 30 years. As we look toward the next 30 years, we will likely face many of the same issues our profession has always faced. We must develop different ways to respond to these issues however, to allow the NP profession to thrive. The key to promoting our profession lies in our zeal to respond to these issues as does flexing our power in numbers. It is vital that every one of us make efforts to promote ourselves and our profession. Focused attention must be made to politicians, health care payers, and most importantly the public. Traditionally, the NP has been hidden behind hospital or practice walls but this has hindered public awareness of our existence and need. We need to quit overlooking the public media who often turn to physicians for expert information on health topics. Historically, NP's have done a poor job promoting the profession as they work so hard to provide quality care to their patients.

3 Steps in Justifying Our Existence

Step One: Know the Facts

Nurses have public respect

A Gallup Poll in November of 2000 discovered that, for the second year in a row, nurses were believed to have the highest standards of honesty and ethics of any other profession by the public. Nearly 80% of the Americans surveyed in this poll said nurses have high ethical standards well ahead of physicians at just over 60%. The empathetic care nurses provide is likely the root cause of the strong respect by the public. Health consumers know they can find a listening ear and helpful hand from a nurse but when this is found from our physician counterparts they are surprised.

NP's provide quality care similar to physicians.

Multiple studies support the quality care nurse
practitioners provide (1-11,15). In a recent study
(published in *JAMA*) 1316 patients were randomly
assigned to either nurse practitioners or physicians. The
study proved that patient outcomes were comparable
(1). In a review of 12 studies, it was found that the
quality of care provided by NP's was higher than that for
physicians on parameters including preventative
actions, patient communication, and reduction in
patients symptoms (15). There has yet to be a study
showing lower quality of care with NP's in comparison to
MD's.

NP's are cost effective.

The cost effectiveness of NP's has been examined many
times as well (15-22). NP's are not only paid less but
they also have found to deliver primary care in a more
cost effective manner than physicians. The
Congressional Office of Technology Assessment after a
review of several studies concluded that NP's can deliver
as much as 80% of the primary care health services, and
up to 90% of the pediatric primary care provided by
primary care physicians, and do it a an equal to or
better quality and at a lower cost (15). The American
Academy of Nurse Practitioner has created a highly
recommended handout documenting the cost
effectiveness of NP's (www.aanp.org).

Patient Satisfaction is high with NP care.

Study after study also documents high satisfaction
ratings with NP provided care (12-15).

Nurse practitioners have been in existence for over 36
years yet many of us still get the question "What is a

nurse practitioner"? Evidence continues to mount that nurse practitioners provide high quality care that is ranked high in patient satisfaction and also cost effective. Our profession receives very little bad press but also very little press of any sort. The problem with the lack of familiarity with our profession lies solely with us. In order for our profession to be recognized we need to begin promoting it. We need to stop hiding behind other professions and organizations and begin to advertise our own profession. Open your local yellow pages and just try to find a nurse practitioner listed.

Step Two: Ensure Recognition

Clarify our role.

We must clarify our role in health care to the public, politicians and health care payers. Consumers are demanding the services we are trained to provide including wellness promotion, illness prevention, personalized education, and empathetic care. We do a great job of providing these services now we need to make it known.

Ensure Reimbursement

Reimbursement is crucial for the future of NP's. The NP role will not survive if there are significant financial barriers. NP's must seek and ensure inclusion on managed care panels and governmental programs. Each one of us should bill directly for our services, rather than through our collaborating physicians so that payers recognize us, and our cost effective, quality care.

Step Three: Provide Outstanding Patient Care

Providing outstanding patient care is what we do best and we must continue to keep our focus on the patient.

It is also imperative that we demonstrate our outstanding care via research. Conducting studies to further provide data to support our claims. Studies should be performed to measure:

-Cost effectiveness of NP provided care

-Quality of NP care provided in a variety of populations and situations (Long-term care, urgent care, etc.)

-Long-term outcomes of NP care such as the morbidity and mortality among common disease states (diabetes, hypertension, etc.)

-The outcomes of preventative care provided by NP's such as whether the risks of developing hypertension or diabetes is reduced when preventative strategies are initiated by NP's

-The effects of collaborative practice arrangements

Barriers to Promotion

Certainly, we do have a few barriers (good excuses) for the lack of significant promotion of our profession.

Lack of Training

Most of our training as nurses and as nurse practitioners has focused on the development of our clinical knowledge and skills with very little (if any) business training. Nurse practitioner programs need to continue to focus their attention on the care of the patient but perhaps begin to include business and marketing courses to give us the business basics to compete in today's health care environment. Those of us who are out of school need to have resources to obtain this information on our own.

Costs

Marketing and promotion can be very expensive. A good ad in the yellow pages can run $500.00 per month. Newspaper ads may cost the same to run an ad for just one day. Cost is a barrier to a profession that does not usually make the decisions with how monies are spent within a practice or organization. Chapter 8 discusses some economical marketing techniques to market both ourselves and thus in return our profession.

Controversy in a name

An old debate surfaces frequently with regard to our title of nurse practitioner. Many hope for a name change because they believe the title does little to distinguish us from other nurses. Others find interest in a name change that may encompass both nurse practitioners and physician assistants. The debate is fueled many times by the titles of physician extender, non-physician provider and midlevel provider that are frequently used by politicians, physicians, and lawyers. These titles are far from "image enhancers" and are usually used in cases where the person is ignorant about what we do. However, is a name change really the answer? Instead of changing our name the real solution to enhancing our image may be "marketing our profession". Only after the role of the NP is clearly defined will the media begin calling NP's for commentary on health care issues.

Individual Solutions to Promoting the NP Profession

1. Be Proactive not Reactive

A proactive approach is needed by each and every nurse practitioner. A proactive approach means that you focus your attention on those things you can do something about. A reactive approach, on the other hand, is focusing on circumstances you have no control over such as the efforts of another profession. The difficulty can be knowing what it is you can and cannot change. This is reflected in the Alcoholics Anonymous prayer;

"Lord, give me the courage to change the things which can and ought to be changed, the serenity to accept the things which cannot be changed, and the wisdom to know the difference."

2. Gain Visibility

Tell everyone you have a conversation with that you are a nurse practitioner.

Believe me I know this becomes a daunting task because you know that this will lead to an explanation of what it is we do. We need to realize, however, that this is the single best thing we can do to promote the nurse practitioner profession. Each person you tell will likely tell several others what you told them (or close to it) about our profession. Keep your explanation short and simple and try refraining from comparisons to other professions such as physicians. Instead, explain our profession as a separate role. At the same time don't be afraid to use the word "nurse." The word "nurse" should not impair our professional image but enhance it. Surveys have shown that nurses are the most trusted health professional and this can be a great quality for someone in the provider role. You may choose to make up your own definition, that of an organization, or even use this one if you would like.

"A nurse practitioner is a registered nurse with additional graduate training which enables them to diagnose and manage acute and chronic illness that may include ordering labs and x-rays and prescribing medications. Nurse practitioners tend to focus on the whole person in preventing illness and promoting wellness."

Volunteer to speak at public health events and write articles for public literary sources.

The media enjoys having guest editorials and articles written by experts. Nurse practitioners are probably not who they turn to first in health related issues but they will if you make yourself known and available to them (especially on a short notice). Start by identifying the reporters in your area who cover health topics for the newspaper, radio, and television. Then make these reporters aware that you are available for quotes on health topics or issues.

3. Support Your Peers

Choose nurse practitioners for yours and your family's health care needs.

We need to make the statement that we prefer to seek the care of nurse practitioners for our own family. Make your decision known to your family, friends, and anyone else you have an opportunity to tell.

Refer to other nurse practitioners

Don't be afraid to send a referral to another nurse practitioner that may practice in a setting or specialty other than your own.

4. Support Nurse Practitioner Organizations and Marketing Campaigns

Joining organizations such as those listed in chapter two allow the expansion of the nurse practitioner profession on a national level. Additional organizations assisting in the marketing of the NP role include:

The National Nurse Practitioner Directory (www.npclinics.com) is a national listing of practicing nurse practitioners. The directory is inexpensive to join and gives the public access to NP's throughout the country.

The National Nurse Practitioner Marketing Campaign is a new effort focused on marketing the profession on a national level. (www.nurse.net)

5. Advertise

Spend a small amount of your own salary advertising. Build a web site, place a yellow page ad, or even donate to a non-profit agency that will advertise your name and your profession. No matter how small, every effort will progress the recognition of the nurse practitioner profession.

1). Mundinger, M., Kane, R., Lenz, E., Totten, A., Tsai, W. et al. (2000). Primary Care Outcomes in Patients Treated by Nurse Practitioners or Physicians: A Randomized Trial. <u>The Journal of the American Medical Foundation, 283, (1).</u> 59-68.

2). Brown, S., Grimes, D. A Meta-analysis of Nurse Practitioners and Nurse Midwifes in Primary Care. *American Nurses Publishing.* Washington, DC, 1993.

3). Schultz, J., et al. Nurse Practitioners' Effectiveness in NICU. *Nursing Management.* 1994;25(10):50-53.

4). Crosby, F., Ventura, M., and Feldman, M. Future Research Recommendations for Establishing Nurse Practitioner Effectiveness. *Nurse Practitioner.* 12:75, 1987.

5). Gabay, M. and Wolfe, S. Encouraging the Use of Nurse-Midwifes: A Report for Policy Makers. *Public Citizens Publication.* Washington, DC. 1995.

6). Prescott, P. and Driscoll, L. Evaluating Nurse Practitioner Performance. *Nurse Practitioner.* 1980;5:28-32.

7). Sacket, D. et al. The Burlington Randomized Trial of the Nurse Practitioner. *N Eng J Med.* 1976; 290:251-156.

8). System Sciences, Inc. Nurse Practitioners and the Physicians Assistant Training and Development Study: Final Report. *Contract No. HRA 230-75-0198.* Bethesda, MD: System Sciences, Inc., September, 1975.

9). Hooker, R. and McCaig, L. Use of Physician Assistants and Nurse Practitioners in Primary Care. *Health Affairs.* 2001; 20(4):231-238.

10). Lee, R., Skelton, R., Skene, C. Routine Neonatal Examination: Effectiveness of Trainee Paediatrician Compared with Advance Practice Neonatal Nurse Practitioner. *Arch Dis Child, Fetal Neonatal Ed.* 2001;85:F100-F104.

11). Aubrey, W. and Yoxall, C. Evaluation of the Role of the Neonatal NP in Resuscitation of Preterm Infants at Birth. *Arch Dis Child, Fetal Neonatal Ed.* 2001:85:F96-99.

12). Rekevics, C., Harte, S., Meyer, K., Shively, M., & Ebersole-Kauffman, D. (1999). Patient Satisfaction with Nurse Practitioners. 1998/99 APN Sourcebook, 14-16.

13). Congressional Budget Office, US Congress. Physicians Extender: Their Current and Future Role in Medical Care Delivery. Washington, DC.: US Governmental Printing Office; April 1979.

14). Kuhl, S. and Clever, L. Acceptance of the Nurse Practitioner. *Am J Nursing.* 1974: 251-256.

15). *Health Technology Case Study 37: Nurse Practitioners, Physician Assistants, and Certified Nurse Midwifes: A Policy Analysis.* Washington DC: US Congress Office of Technology Assessment; December 1986; 39. Government Printing Office Publication OTA-HCS-37.

16). Nichols, L. Estimating Costs of Underused Advanced Practice Nurses. *Nursing Economics.* 1992;10(5):343-351.

17). Burl, J., et al. Demonstration of the Cost-Effectiveness of a Nurse Practitioner/Physician Team in Long-Term Care Facilities. *HMO Practice*. 1994;9(4):157-161.

18). Frampton, J., Wall, S. Exploring the Use of NP's and PA's in Primary Care. *HMO Practice*. 1994;8(4):165-170.

19). Scweitzer, S: The Relative Costs of Physicians and New Health Practitioners. In Staffing Primary Care in 1990: Physician Replacement and Cost Savings. Springer, New York, 1991.

20). Greenfield, S., et al. Efficiency and Cost of Primary Care of Nurses and Physician Assistants. *N Engl J Med*. 1978;298(305).

21). Robyn, D. and Hadley, J. National Health Insurance and the New Health Occupations: Nurse Practitioners and Physicians Assistants. *Journal of Health Politics, Policy, and Law*. 5(3);1980:451.

22). Smith, K. Health Practitioners: Efficient Utilization and Cost of Health Care.

About the Author

Dr. Kevin Letz is a practicing nurse practitioner at The Allergy and Asthma Center in Fort Wayne, Indiana. He received his nurse doctorate (N.D.) degree from Rush University in Chicago, Illinois, masters of science in nursing (M.S.N.) from The University of Saint Francis in Fort Wayne, Indiana and his bachelor of science (B.S.N.) and associate of science in nursing (A.D.N.) at Purdue University in Indiana. Dr. Letz is board certified as a family nurse practitioner, adult nurse practitioner, and pediatric nurse practitioner and as an emergency nurse. Dr. Letz is owner of PreviCare Consulting and is available for lectures. He can be contacted by mail at Previcare, Inc., 2602 Barry Knoll Way, Fort Wayne, IN. 46845

Appendix A: Estimate of Nurse Practitioner Worth ® (examples in parenthesis)

Number of work days {52 weeks x (5) work days=
____(260) days – vacation days ____ (15) – sick days___ (5)
– conference days ____(5) = total work days____ (235)}

A._____ (235)

X

Number of visits per day { NP's average 15-20 per day, A new NP may start at 10 patient visits per day, What do you feel comfortable with, What is expected of you, What are other in the practice doing}

_____ (20) = B. _____(4700)

X

Average cost per visit {Ask or research to find the most frequently billed CPT code for the practice and the amount billed to that CPT code}

_____ ($40) = C._____(188,000)

X

% of reimbursement by the practice {Ask the office manager or billing specialist at the office. 80-90% is considered a very good reimbursement percentage}

_____ (90% or 0.90) = D._____ (169,200)

X

Overhead costs (30-40% solo-physician practice, 15-30% multi-physician practice, includes building, insurance, staff, supplies, utilities etc.)

_____ **(30% or 0.30)   = E._____ (50,760)**

D. _____(169,200) minus E._____ (50,760) =
$_____ ($118,000) Total Revenue

Appendix B: Sample Employment Contract

Employment Contract

THIS AGREEMENT, made and entered into this___day of, _____ (year), by and between _____, of _____ (city), _____ (state) (hereinafter "Corporation) and _____, N.P., a nurse practitioner qualified to provide services in _____ (state), (hereinafter "Nurse Practitioner.

WHEREAS, Nurse Practitioner desires to provide nursing services as an employee of the Corporation; and

WHEREAS, the Corporation has determined that in the interest of the Corporation's business, it is desirable to employ Nurse Practitioner for his/her professional abilities and skills.

NOW THEREFORE, for and in consideration of the mutual covenants and agreements herein set out, the parties mutually agree as follow:

EMPLOYMENT. The Corporation hereby employs Nurse Practitioner, and Nurse Practitioner accepts such employment, for the provision of nursing services as defined in "Exhibit A, Nurse Practitioner Job Description" attached hereto and incorporated herein by reference (hereinafter "Nursing Services") on behalf of the Corporation, subject to the supervision and direction of the Corporation and subject to the laws and regulations of the State of _____.

**TERM OF EMPLOYMENT. The term of this Agreement
shall begin on the _____day of _____(month),
_____(year), and shall have a term of _____ calendar
months. This agreement is subject to all rights of
termination prior to its expiration date as provided
herein, and if no termination occurs, the Corporation
and Nurse Practitioner may at the conclusion of the
initial term, extend this Agreement for annual periods.**

**DUTIES OF NURSE PRACTITIONER. The Nurse
Practitioner acknowledges and agrees to provide nursing
services as set forth in exhibit A, on behalf of the
corporation. Although the Nurse Practitioner shall be a
salaried employee it is agreed upon that an average work
week will be 45 hours.**

**COMPENSATION. As compensation for Nursing Services
provided pursuant to this Agreement, the Corporation
shall pay to Nurse Practitioner and annual salary in an
amount of $_____ per year. The Nurse
Practitioners salary shall be prorated and paid twice per
month on the day established by the Corporation, with
the compensation paid for the first and last payroll
period to be prorated if necessary.**

**PRODUCTIVITY COMPENSATION. As an incentive to the
Nurse Practitioner, the Corporation will automatically
increase the Nurse Practitioner's base salary after the
following criteria have been satisfied:**

a. No salary increase for the first ___ months .

**b. After ___ months and seeing ___ patients per week for
one (1) month the Nurse Practitioner's salary will
increase to $_____ per year.**

**c. After seeing ___ patients per week for one (1) month
the Nurse Practitioner's base salary will be increased to
$ _____ per year.**

d. In addition to the base salary provided above, Corporation shall pay to Nurse Practitioner for the first twelve (12) month period of the term and for each successive twelve (12) month period thereafter, productivity compensation. The productivity compensation shall be equal to ten percent (10%) of Nurse Practitioner's gross compensation over $200,000.00 for each twelve (12) month period.

For purpose of this Agreement, "Nurse Practitioner's Gross Production" shall mean the total amount of professional fees generated by or attributable to Nurse Practitioner's production and actually collected and received by Employer during such twelve (12) month period, as determined by the Corporation in its sole discretion. In determining what amount or percentage of the total capitation payments received by Nurse Practitioner from health maintenance or similar organization will take into consideration Nurse Practitioner's productivity and efficiency in working within the payment system established by such health maintenance or organization by Corporation. Corporation shall pay the amount due to Nurse Practitioner under the terms of this paragraph for each such twelve (12) month period (net of required withholdings and deductions) within thirty (30) days after the end of each such twelve (12) month period. In the event the Nurse Practitioner disagrees with the amount of any productivity payment, Nurse Practitioner shall give written notice thereof to Corporation no later than thirty (30) days after the date of such payment.

BENEFITS. Nurse Practitioner shall be entitled to the following benefits while agreement remains in effect:

a. Corporation will pay the Nurse Practitioner's license fees as a Registered Nurse and Nurse Practitioner and fees for obtainment and renewal of Prescriptive Authority.

b. The Corporation shall pay conference fees and associated cost for the Nurse Practitioner's continuing education which is reasonably required to maintain Nurse Practitioner's license as a Registered Nurse and Nurse Practitioner, provided that such education is approved by the Corporation in advance and not to exceed $ _____ per calendar year. This amount may also be used for annual subscriptions and educational material for the Nurse Practitioner.

c. The Nurse Practitioner and the Nurse Practitioner's immediate family (Limited to the Nurse Practitioner's spouse and dependant children living at home) shall receive full coverage of health, vision, and dental insurance.

d. ___weeks paid vacation, ___paid personal days, and ___paid sick days per twelve (12) month period. Vacation and personal days will be used during the contract period only. Sick days may be carried forward up to a maximum of ___days.

e. Corporation will provide the Nurse Practitioner with _____weeks paid time to attend continuing education events and in-services.

f. Corporation will provide Nurse Practitioner with malpractice insurance as a Nurse Practitioner.

g. $_____term live insurance coverage if Employee qualifies for non-smoking rates. This policy will be provided by the company of the Corporation's choice.

h. Enrollment in the Employer's 401k plan.

TERMS OF AGREEMENT. This agreement may be terminated at any time during the initial term of any extended term by the mutual agreement of the parties, by the death of Nurse Practitioner, or voluntarily by either party providing written notice to the other party at least thirty (30) days before the effective date of termination. In the event this Agreement is terminated by notice without cause, Nurse Practitioner, if requested by Corporation, shall continue to provide services during the thirty (30) day period and shall be paid her/his salary for the days the Nurse Practitioner provides services. Corporation may elect to terminate the employment of Nurse Practitioner and terminate the services of Nurse Practitioner by paying the Nurse Practitioner her/his salary for the thirty (30) days period.

In addition, this agreement may be terminated at any time during the term or any extended term by Corporation "for cause". For purposes of this section, termination of Nurse Practitioner "for cause" shall include the default by Nurse Practitioner in any term of this Agreement and further shall include the following:

a. Nurse Practitioner becoming disqualified to render services within the state;

b. Nurse Practitioner engaging in any conduct which is unethical under the code of ethics either of the American Nurses Association or _____ State Nurses Association.

c. Nurse Practitioner's personal use of alcohol, narcotics, or other drugs to the detriment of Corporation or any of its patients or resulting in his/her inability to perform his/her duties under this agreement.

In the event of termination by Corporation "for cause" the employment relationship shall terminate immediately upon delivery of written notice to Nurse Practitioner. Nurse Practitioner shall receive salary due him/her as of the effective date of termination.

In the event Nurse Practitioner dies, retires, or is determined to be disabled, such event shall terminate the employment relationship and Nurse Practitioner shall be entitled to his/her salary to the date of death, retirement or determination of disability.

RESTRICTIVE COVENANT. In consideration of employment, Nurse Practitioner agrees to be bound by this non-competition provision. In the event of Nurse Practitioner's termination of employment "for cause", Nurse Practitioner agrees that he/she shall not, either during, or at any time within two (2) years after any such termination of his/her employment, either solicit employment of be employed or self-employed, either directly or indirectly, whether as an employee, sole proprietor, joint venture, partner, shareholder, or independent contractor, by any person, group, entity or practice, or in any capacity of the type and character in the practice of _____ within a 20 mile radius of the Corporation's practice facility. Nurse Practitioner acknowledges and agrees that the above-referenced area is the service area of the Corporation. Nurse Practitioner further acknowledges and agrees that this restrictive covenant is a reasonable restriction and necessary for the protection of Corporation's legitimate business interests.

Nurse Practitioner recognizes and agrees that in the event Nurse Practitioner violates the provisions of this Section, it will be difficult to compensate Corporation with monetary damages and that the Corporation will suffer irreparable damage. Nurse Practitioner will be liable to Corporation for any damages to the Corporation as a direct results of the Nurse Practitioner's breach of this Section and the costs and Corporation's attorney fees.

CONFIDENTIALITY. Corporation and Nurse Practitioner agree that Corporation maintains certain nonpublic, confidential and proprietary information (hereinafter referred to as "Confidential Information"), to which

Nurse Practitioner, as an employee, has access. Corporation and Nurse Practitioner acknowledge and agree that this is in the best interest of Corporation and all employees to maintain the proprietary and confidentiality of such Confidential Information for the benefit of the medical practice and its owners. "Confidential Information" for purposes of this section and this Agreement shall mean and include patient lists, schedule of patients, contracts, managed care contracts, payer agreements, financial statements, compensation formulas, compensation amounts for employees, strategic planning documents, and all minutes of committee meetings together with such other documents and information Corporation may designate and stamp or mark as "Confidential Information." Nurse Practitioner covenants and agrees that during the term of this Agreement, she will protect the Confidential Information of the Corporation and will not discuss, disclose or divulge Confidential Information to any persons other than professionals serving or engaged by Corporation. Further, Nurse Practitioner agrees that in the event her employment terminates with Corporation for any reason, Nurse Practitioner agrees to return to Corporation any and all Confidential Information in her possession, to include any notes and/or memoranda deriving information from Confidential Information.

GOVERNING STATE. This agreement has been executed in the state of _____ and shall be enforceable only in the state and federal courts of said state. This Agreement is to be construed in accordance with the laws of the state.

COVERAGE. In the Nurse Practitioner's absence, incapacity, infirmity or emergency the Corporation shall arrange for medical coverage of the Nurse Practitioner.

ASSIGNMENT. The parties agree that this Agreement is personal to the Nurse Practitioner and Corporation and cannot be assigned by either party without the written mutual consent of the other.

MERGER OF NEGOTIATIONS. It is agreed that this Agreement as a whole constitutes the entire Agreement of employment between the Corporation and Nurse Practitioner. There is no statement, promise, agreement, or obligation in existence, which may conflict with the terms of this Agreement or may modify, enlarge, or invalidate this Agreement or any provisions hereof.

SURVIVAL OF COVENANTS. This Agreement shall be binding upon any successors or heirs or personal representatives of the parties hereto. The covenants shall survive any termination or rescission of the Agreement unless the Corporation executes a written agreement specifically releasing Nurse Practitioner from such covenants.

CONSTRUCTION. Throughout this Agreement, the use of the singular number shall be construed to include the plural, then singular, and the use of any gender shall include all genders, whenever required by the context.

IN WITNESS WHEREOF, the Corporation and Nurse Practitioner have entered into this Agreement on the day and year first above written.

Executed this ____ day of _____, _____.

Corporation:_____

Business address:

Nurse Practitioner:_____

Home address:

Witness:_____

Appendix C: Nurse Practitioner Job Description

Nurse Practitioner Job Description

Position Summary:

Works independently, but under the supervision of a physician to provide patient care, educate patients and families, and act as a resource staff.

Reports to:

Administratively: _____

Medically: _____

Specific Responsibilities:

Comprehensive Physical Assessment of Patients.

1). Review patient records to determine health status.

2). Take patient history, including physical, developmental and psychosocial health status.

3). Perform complete physical examinations.

4). Perform developmental screening examination on children.

5). Document appropriate patient/family information and/or health appraisal data.

Establish Medical Diagnosis for Short Term or Chronic Health Problems.

1). Evaluate patient presentation and establish diagnosis.

2). Assess psychosocial, cognitive, and personal assets and limitations of patient/ family and plan care to incorporate those needs.

Determine Learning Needs of Patients.

1). Develop individualized teaching plans with the client based on covert health needs.

2). Counsel individuals, families, and groups about health and illness and promote health maintenance.

3). Recognize, develop, and implement professional community education programs related to health care.

Order and Interpret Lab Tests (including diagnostic and invasive procedures).

1). Request commonly performed initial and follow up lab, radiological, and other diagnostic studies, including isotopic, histologic, computerized, and other studies.

2). Order lab procedures.

3). Order/perform venipuncture to obtain blood samples.

4). Interpret studies performed/ordered.

5). Inform patient/family of planned procedures and treatments.

Prescribing Drugs.

1). Prescribing oral, parenteral, intramuscular, or subcutaneous medications under conditions in Nurse Practitioner agreement with Medical Director.

2). Regulate medication dosage.

3). Controlled substances may be dispensed.

Perform Therapeutic or Corrective Measures

1). Assess and manage surgical wounds, necrotic lesions, decubitus, leg ulcers, etc.

2). Repair and treat lacerations.

3). Control external hemorrhage.

4). Apply dressing and bandages.

5). Administer medications and intravenous fluids.

6). Remove superficial foreign bodies.

7). Carry out aseptic and isolation techniques.

8). Provide emergency care in accordance with CPR/ACLS protocols.

Refer patients to Appropriate Licensed Physician or Other Healthcare Providers.

1). Screen patients to determine need for medical attention.

2). Referrals to community agencies, services, and providers, as necessary, to meet home care needs or other expertise required.

3). Arrange for, or refer patients to needed services that cannot be provided at the facility.

Records Management.

1). Initiate and maintain accurate records, appropriate legal documents, and other health and nursing care reports.

2). Participate in the development, execution, and periodic review of the written policies governing the services that the medical facility furnishes.

3). Participate with physicians in periodic review of the patients' health records.

4). Assure that adequate patient health records are maintained and transferred as required when patients are referred.

5). Participate in periodic and joint evaluation of services rendered, including, but not limited to, chart reviews, patient evaluations, and case outcome statistics.

6). Participate in the joint review and revision of adopted protocols for medical care plans.

Medical Support for the Nurse Practitioner:

The Nurse Practitioner will function according to the guidelines of state statutes, rules and regulations given the following acts of supervision by the Medical Director or his/her physician designees:

Consulting the Physician.

Should the Nurse Practitioner consult a physician regarding a particular patient, either by telephone or in person, for any condition, orders may be received and relayed to the patient. In this case, documentation in the chart is required. This indicates a physician was consulted and specified orders received.

Medications.

Although Nurse Practitioners may prescribe medications, there must be a collaborative agreement with the physician. Physician review of Nurse Practitioner documentation and prescription practices will be ongoing with at least 5% random sampling of charts.

Record Review.

Charts of patients seen by the Nurse Practitioner may be reviewed and signed by the Medical Director and/or his/her medical designees. Content of documentation should be checked for adherence to standard practices.

Coverage.

In his/her absence, the Medical Director shall arrange for medical coverage for the Nurse Practitioner.

Appendix D: Sample Collaborative Practice Agreement

THIS PRACTICE AGREEMENT is made and entered into this ___ day of _____, year _____, by and among the advanced practice nurse, _____ (hereinafter "NP") and the below licensed physician(s), to be effective upon the granting of prescriptive authority to the Nurse Practitioner by the State Board of Nursing.

WITNESSETH:

WHEREAS, the purpose of this Practice Agreement is to set forth, in writing, the manner in which NP and the licensed physician(s) as provided hereunder shall cooperate, coordinate, and consult with each other in the provision of health care to patients; and

WHEREAS, this agreement sets forth provisions for the type of collaboration between or among the NP and the licensed physician(s) and the reasonable and timely review by the licensed physician(s) of the prescribing practices of the NP.

NOW, THEREFORE in consideration of the mutual covenants, agreements and conditions hereinafter set forth, the parties hereto agree as follows:

Addresses. Below appears a complete list of names, home, and business addresses, zip codes, and telephone numbers of the licensed physician(s) and the NP.

Name M.D.

Home Address

Phone

Professional Address

Name N.P.

Home Address

Phone

Professional Address

Specialty Board Certification. All specialty board certifications of the licensed physician(s) and NP are set forth hereunder.

Physician Name   **Specialty Board Certification**

N.P. Name   **Specialty Board Certification**

Purpose. The Practice Agreement is a means of communicating, in writing, the prescribing environment between or among the NP and the licensed physician(s) (hereinafter "MD(s)") pursuant to State Board of Nursing requirements. This Practice Agreement sets forth the manner of collaboration between NP and MD(s), including how the NP and MD(s) work together, share practice trends and responsibilities, maintain geographic proximity, and provide coverage during absence, incapacity, infirmity, or emergency by the licensed practitioner.

Nature of Collaborative Practice. The MD(s) and the NP shall collaborate in the management of family practice patients. The MD(s) have an office at _____, and have privileges at _____. The NP is an employee at _____, and his/her responsibility in the collaborative practice will be to work with the MD(s) through protocols and consultation and act in accordance with this Practice Agreement for prescriptive authority. For a more detailed description of the collaboration, cooperation, and coordination between or among the NP and MD(s) see Job Description, attached hereto, incorporated herein, and marked as "Exhibit A."

Geographic proximity is assured by virtue of the fact that the MD(s) and the NP share the same office facilities. The MD(s) shall be available to the NP to provide consultation and patient assessment as needed. Such availability shall include but be limited to electronic means or backup MD(s). The NP's prescriptive privileges will not extend beyond the MD(s) scope or practice. The NP will not be expected to perform services outside the traditional role described for a NP pursuant to state law and regulations.

Limitations of NP's Prescriptive Authority. The collaborating MD(s) have limited the NP prescriptive authority to drug schedules 3, 3 narcotic, 4 and 5.

Review Process. The NP shall submit documentation of the NP's prescribing practices to the MD(s) within seven (7) days. Documentation of prescribing practices shall include, but not be limited to, at least 5 percent (5%) sampling of charts and medications prescribed for patients.

Duration and Termination. This Practice Agreement will remain in force as long as the MD(s) and the NP engage in collaborative management of patient care as described herein. Should there be any changes to this Practice Agreement including changes in the prescriptive authority of the collaborating MD(s), the State Board of Nursing shall be notified and a new practice agreement must be submitted to the State Board of Nursing for approval. This agreement shall automatically terminate if the NP or MD(s) no longer have an active, unrestricted license.

Appendix E: Estimating Expenses in an Independent NP Practice

	Monthly Costs
Staffing	
1 RN	_____ ($2700)
1 Office Staff	_____ (2080)
Office Space	
Rent	_____ (2500)
Renovation	_____ (200)
Utilities	
Water	_____ (100)
Garbage	_____ (50)
Electric	_____ (250)
Telephone	_____ (300)
(3 lines, pager, cell phone, internet)	
Cleaning/Maintenance	_____ (350)
Hazardous Waste	_____ (100)
Supplies/Equipment	
Medical	_____ (600)

Business Essentials for Nurse Practitioners

Office	_____	(400)
Professional		
Malpractice Insurance	_____	(100)
Health Insurance	_____	(750)
Disability Insurance	_____	(0)
Continuing Education	_____	(150)
Accounting	_____	(100)
Legal Fees	_____	(50)
Licenses/Memberships	_____	(50)
Bank Fees	_____	(25)
Physician Collaboration Fees	_____	(400)
Building Insurance	_____	(100)
Other		
Subscriptions	_____	(25)
Auto	_____	(300)
Promotion/Advertising	_____	(250)
Other	_____	( )
Total Monthly Costs =	_____	($10,000)

Appendix F: Sample Business Plan

Business Plan for N. P.

Executive Summary

Company: The Wellness Practitioners
Primary Care with a Holistic Approach

Current status: Planning and initial preparation.

Products/Services: Primary care with a holistic and individualized approach.

Description of our market: Maintenance of wellness and adjunctive treatment of illness.

Company objectives: Develop a well-respected clinic providing primary care to individuals who are interested in combining traditional and non-traditional medicine.

Funding plans: Seeking 40,000.00 start up fees.

History and Position to Date

Introduction to Your Business

Why business will succeed: The Wellness Practitioner's specialize in you. Individualized health care is what we are about. We recognize the fact that everyone's health needs are different and we work with you to optimize your total health.

Company vision:
The provision of holistic and individualized primary health care to all populations.

Short-term goals: Build a well-known and well-respected organization, which assists individuals in optimizing health and wellness.

Company values: Trust, Relationship building, Caring.

Business Structure

S-Corporation

Reason for this structure: Allows for the greatest growth.

Management Team

My experience: Management of health care professionals, Experience in marketing in the medical field, Extensive experience in working with patients in multiple health care settings.

My skills/qualifications: Board certification as a family nurse practitioner, Masters of science degree in nursing, Extensive health care experience in multiple areas, Managerial experience in medical surgical department.

Other key personnel: Registered Nurse, Office Manager.

Products and Services

Providing primary care, which focuses on health prevention and taking a holistic and individualized approach.

Steps required to make product ready for market: Establish office setting and hire staff.

Cost to make product ready for market: $20,000.00.

Time until ready for market: 2 months.

Market differentiation: A professional, caring atmosphere devoted to providing individualized care.

Practitioners who take a holistic and preventative approach to medical care.

Possible new or complementary products: Complimentary health care modalities.

Regulatory issues: Permit.

Market Research

Customers

Geographic scope: Northern Small Town, USA.

Customer needs: All individuals seeking a primary care provider with an interest in them and willingness to consider alternative modalities.

Market growth: Continued growth as baby boomers age.

Growth relative to local economy: Well.

Demographics: Middle age, female, middle class, married.

Product Features

Feature: Individualized primary health care.

Benefit to customer: Individualized medical care both preventative and holistic in nature.

Proof: Several studies showing both the quality of care Nurse Practitioners provide and high patient satisfaction ratings.

Feature: Preventative approach to care.

Benefit to customer: Improvement in total health.

Feature: Holistic approach to care.

Benefit to customer: Care, which is focused on both the body and the mind and is all encompassing.

Customer Sensitivities

Quality, Appearance, Customer service, Operating characteristics, Reputation, Advertising and promotion, Employee attitude or appearance.

Competitors

Family practice physicians, Chiropractors and alternative health care providers.

Competitors' products: Well established businesses versus a new but knowledgeable start up.

Strengths and weaknesses, relative to us: Unwillingness to consider alternative health modalities. Well-established business, which are bringing in money. Limited marketing and advertising.

Critical factors for success: Maintain customers.
Develop a customer base.
Develop respect from medical community.
Market to key people.

Business Strategy

Pricing Policy

Pricing factors: Consumer Perceptions, Business Conditions, Channels of Distribution, and Production Capacity.

Advertising and Promotion

Long-term promotional goals: To be a well-respected holistic primary care center.

Short-term promotional goals: Direct advertising to key influencers in the medical arena.

Marketing message: Select a primary care specialist interested in you and willing to use complimentary treatment.

Media: Mailings to key individuals, which do not require a large budget. Newspaper advertisements in order to reach a large volume of people.

Monitoring marketing effectiveness: Track return on investment by asking patients how they heard about us.

Promotional budget: 5,000.00

Location

Factors in choosing location: Convenient location in a highly populated community setting.

Competitive advantages: Ease of access and improved visibility.

Operations

Sales and Sales Management

Who will conduct sales: All employees.

Training: Internal.

Incentives: Employees will receive recruitment bonuses.

Customer complaints: Speak and listen to them directly and institute a tracking system to assess reoccurrence.

Manufacturing/Supply

Materials/supplies needed: Two employees. Medical and office equipment.

Vendor(s): Large medical supply companies and office supply companies to obtain lowest costs.

Terms of sale: Reduced cost to our company for bulk volume of ordering.

Staffing Issues

Key positions: Registered nurse with office experience to provide patient care including education, history taking, medication administration, immunization, assistance with procedures, phlebotomy and telephone triaging.
Office manager to assist with patient check in and check out, billing and appointment scheduling.

Recruitment: Word of mouth.

Dress code: Professional scrubs purchased by the corporation.

Forecasting

Financial Statements
Attached.

Sensitivity Analysis

Financing Requirements

Funds required: $20,000.00

Use of funds:
Establish office location = $2,000.00
First month staff salary = $5,000.00
Advertising and promotion = $5,000.00
Supplies and equipment = $8,000.00

Money from partners, investors: $5,000.00

Desired funding sources: Small business loans.

When needed: This month

Business Controls

Accounting System: Quick Books Pro

Reason for choice: Ease of use and familiar with all accountants.

Auditors: Outside coding specialists.

Sales monitoring: Computer aided sales and inventory monitoring.

Marketing records: New buyer tracking.

Customer feedback/complaints: Customer satisfaction is essential to have returning customers and attain customer referrals.

Appendix G: Press Release Sample

For Immediate Release

Area NP to Speak in Reno, Nevada

Dr. Kevin Letz will speak for the second year in a row at the annual meeting of The American Academy of Nurse Practitioners. Dr. Letz's lecture entitled "What's Now and What's Coming in Allergy and Asthma Treatment Modalities" will overview current and up and coming therapies in the treatment of allergic disease and asthma. The rate of allergic disease and asthma has increased substantially over the last decade, which has prompted the discovery of new treatment options and the improvement of therapies that have been available.

Dr. Letz is considered an expert in this area and currently functions as one of the nurse practitioner providers at The Allergy and Asthma Center in Fort Wayne. There has been a considerable expansion of nurse practitioners in this specialty not unlike other specialties where the supply of specialty trained physicians is unable to keep up with the demand of the public.

Appendix H: "Superbill" Sample

Nurse Practitioner Sample, Inc.
1900 Happy Practitioner Place, Fort Wayne, In 46845

Patient Name: MR#:
Guarantor:
Address: Date:

Diagnosis:

_____   _____   _____

__ Health supervision V20.2

Office Services: Fee_____

__ New patient __ 99202 __ 99203 __ 99204 __ 99205

__ Est. patient __ 99211 __ 99212 __ 99213 __ 99214 __ 99215
Procedures: Fee_____

__ Phlebotomy 99195 __ Lesion removal 17110

__ Vaccine administration 90472
Laboratory: Fee_____

__ CBC w/plt. 85023 __ Glucose 82947

__ Mono test 86308 __ Throat culture 87081
Injections: Fee_____

__ Allergy 95115 __ Pneumovax 90732

__ Ampicillin 250mg 90788 __ Other:

Total Charges   _____

Total Paid   _____
        Cash ___ Check #_____
        Charge: Visa___ MasterCard___ Discover___
Date of next appointment: _____
Services Rendered by: Nurse Practitioner, NP

Appendix I: E&M Clinical Examples of Established Patients

99211

An office visit for a teenager for removal of sutures placed in the ER 7 days ago.

An office visit for a 30-year-old patient requesting a return to work slip.

An office visit for an 80-year-old patient for her monthly B-12 injection by the nurse.

99212

An office visit for a teenager with contusions and abrasions after a skateboarding fall.

An office visit for a college student with complaints of a sore throat, fever and fatigue.

An office visit for a child returning for follow-up after a recent otitis media.

99213

An office visit for a child on prn bronchodilators for exercise induced asthma.

An office visit with a 50-year-old for adjustment of hypertension medications.

An office visit with a elderly patient with IDDM and CAD for regular monitoring.

99214

An office visit with a 20-year-old female patient with new onset RLQ abdominal pain.

An office visit with an elderly male patient with benign prostatic hypertrophy and severe bladder outlet obstruction, to discuss further treatment.

An office visit with a child who is presenting with acute dermatitis covering greater than 80 percent of his body.

99215

An office visit with an 80-year old with new onset syncopal episodes.

An office visit with a 30-year-old male with a history of stable schizophrenia who is currently complaining of auditory hallucinations.

An office visit with an 8-year-old patient with newly diagnosed common variable immune deficiency with recommendation for new therapy including intravenous gamma globulin infusions.

Sample Documentation

99212 Established problem focused outpatient office visit

S: Headache right temporal area started 2 days ago. No relief with ibuprofen or aspirin. Pounding in nature. Pain similar to migraine at beginning of the year.
O: Awake, alert, oriented x3, cranial nerves II-XII grossly intact, gait steady, Temp 98.6F, HR 88, RR 20.
A: Classic migraine intractable 346.01
P: Sumatriptan 6mg injection sq now, Sumatriptan 50mg po prn x1, may repeat dose after 2 hours x1

99214 Established Detailed office visit

CC: Headache

HPI: Patient developed pain to frontal area of head 12 days ago. Describes pain as a pressure which is relieved slightly with pressure to forehead or when taking over the counter decongestants. Pain worsens when bending over. Pain is moderately severe and is similar to when she has had previous episodes of sinusitis. Pain is constant but is worse when lying down or with movement.
ROS:
Constitutional: Moderate fatigue, continuous headache, occasional dizziness, no change is appetite or activity level
Eyes: No decreased vision or blurring, no visual auras
Ears/Nose/Throat/Sinus: No change in hearing, mild sore throat from drainage, constant post nasal drip, no sneezing, no ear popping, pain or discharge
Respiratory: Mild cough, no chest pain, no shortness of breath, no wheezing
Cardiovascular: No chest pain, no swelling to extremities

Neurological: Mild dizziness on occasion, no loss of consciousness, no memory or mood changes except feeling "irritable", no numbness, tingling or loss of sensation to extremities

PMH: 10 sinusitis episodes over the last year treated with antibiotics at urgent care clinics, no previous surgeries, "mild hypertension" 4 years ago, P 1 G 1, last visit to clinic was 3 years ago

Social Hx: Married, 1 12 yr old son, non-smoker, 1-2 alcohol drinks per week, denies other illicit drug use

Family Hx: Dad has allergies and hypertension, Mom has history of hysterectomy

Physical:
VS: T 99.9 P 88 B/P 184/98 Wt 224 Ht 5 ft 6 in

Eyes: Visual fields intact, pupils equal, round and reactive to light, ophthalmoscope exam reveals no papillary edema, optic disc sharp

Ears, Nose, Mouth, Throat, Sinus: TM's intact and pearly gray with good light reflection, no ear drainage, nose is patent with red and swollen turbinates, mucopurulent nasal drainage bilaterally, dentition intact, no lesions to mouth or throat, cobble stoning to oropharnyx, mild tonsilar hypertrophy, tenderness to maxillary and frontal sinus areas bilaterally

Respiratory: Respirations regular, even, and easy, Chest clear to auscultation

Cardiovascular: S1S2 regular rate and rhythm with no murmurs gallops or rubs, strong radial and pedal pulses, no peripheral edema, extremities pink, and warm

Neuro: Alert to person, place, and time, Rhomberg test normal, Cranial nerves II-XII grossly intact

GI: Abdomen soft, nontender, no liver or spleen enlargement, bowel sounds intact all 4 quadrants

Assessment: Headache, Acute and chronic sinusitis, high blood pressure reading, vertigo

Plan:
Obtain records from urgent care centers
Review previous medical records from prior visits

Order CT scan of sinus cavities
Initiate antibiotic, nasal corticosteroid, nasal irrigations
Refer to allergist
Lifestyle/dietary recommendations for elevated blood
pressure
Check blood pressure daily and log to bring to next visit
Return next week for follow up visit to check blood
pressure and ensure headache relief
Call if worse or any change in symptoms
Call if not improved in 5 days

Appendix J: Evaluation & Management Worksheet

HISTORY

HPI (History of Present Illness) elements:
__Location __Quality __Severity __Duration __Timing __Context
__Modifying factors __Associated S/S
Brief 1-3 Limited 1-3 Expanded >4 Detailed >4 Comprehensive >4

ROS (Review of systems) elements:
__Constitutional __Eyes __ Ears, nose, throat, mouth __Cardio
__Resp __GI __GU __MS __Skin __Neuro __Psych __Endo
__Hem/Lymph __Immuno
Brief 0 Limited 1 sys. Expanded >2 Detailed 2-9 Compr. >10
PFSH
__Past medical history __Past social history __Family history
Brief 0 Limited 0 Expanded >1 Detailed 3 Compr. 3

EXAMINATION

Constitutional: __Any 3 vital signs __General appearance
Eyes: __Conjunctiva & eyelids __Pupils & Irises __Optic discs
ENT: __Exter. ears & nose __TM's & EAC's __Hearing __Oropharynx
__Nasal mucosa, septum & turbinates __Lips, gums, & teeth
Neck: __Neck __Thyroid
Resp: __Effort __Percussion __Palpation __Auscultation
Cardio: __Heart palp. __Auscultation __Carotid __Abd. Aorta
__Femoral __Pedal pulses __Extremity edema & varicosities
Chest: __Breast inspec. __Palpation breasts & axilla
GI: __Tenderness & masses __liver & spleen __Hernia __Anus,
rectum, perineal __occult stool
GU: MALE: __Scrotal contents __Penis __Prostate
FEMALE: __extern. genitalia __Urethra __Bladder __Cervix __Uterus
__Adnexa & parametria
Lymph: __Neck nodes __Axillae nodes __Groin nodes __Other
MS: __Gait & station __Digits & nails __Joints, bones, muscles in
at least 1 area to include inspection &/or palpation, ROM,
Stability, and strength & tone: __head&neck __spine, ribs, pelvis
__RUE __LUE __ RLE __ LLE
Brief 1 bullet any system/area Limited >6 any sys/area
Expanded >12 from >2 sys/area Detailed >18 from >9 sys/area
Compr. >18 from >9 sys/area

Business Essentials for Nurse Practitioners 201

DECISION MAKING (Need to meet 2 of 3 below)

DIAGNOSIS

_Minor problem (1 point) _Minor problem (1) _Est. prob. stable (1) _Est. prob. Stable (1) _Est. prob. worse (2) _Est. prob. worse (2) _New prob. stable (3) _New prob. further eval. (4) ____

Brief >=1 Limited >=1 Expanded >=2 Detailed >=3 Compr. >=4

DATA

Order/study labs = 1 point Order/study x-ray = 1 Order/study medical tests = 1 Discuss results w/ testing provider = 1 Order old record/added history = 1 Summary of review of old records/additional history = 2 View x-ray, tracing, slide prep by other provider = 2 Total___

Brief >=1 point Limited >=1 Expanded >=2 Detailed >=3 Compr. >=4

RISK

Brief >=minimal Limited >=Limited Expanded >=Moderate Detailed >= Moderate Expanded =High

Must meet requirements for all 3 areas (history, exam, and decision making) in order to justify level of E&M service

Business Essentials for Nurse Practitioners 202

Established Patient – Office – Outpatient

Must meet 2 of 3 Components

Levels	99211	99212	99213	99214	99215
History					
CC	1	1	1	1	1
HPI		1-3	1-3	>=4	>=4
ROS	0	1	1	2-9	>=10
PFSH				1 area	2
Exam					
PE	0 bullets	1-5	6-11	12	18
Decision Making					
DX		Min	Lim	Mult	Ext
Data	None	None-Min	Lim	Mod	Ext
Risk	None	Min	Low	Mod	High

2 of 3 must be met or exceeded

Time
May override other components if >50% of time is counseling

Minutes	5	10	15	25	40

Appendix K: Chart Audit Tool

Provider Name: _____ **Patient Name:** _____

Date of service: _____ **Reviewed by:** _____

Documents Reviewed:

__Medical Record ____Patient Accounts Record
__HCFA 1500 ____Procedure Note

Billed CPT_____ **Correctly coded?** __Yes __No

Medically Necessary? __Yes __No

Comments:
_____
_____

ICD-9 Code Billed_____ **Correctly coded?** __Yes __No

Comments:

_____

_____

Appendix L: History & Physical Documentation

HISTORY-SUBJECTIVE DATA
REVIEW OF SYSTEMS

ID
age, sex, DOB

CC
reason for seeking care

HPI
O-onset
L-location
D-duration
C-character
A-aggravating/associated factors
R-relieving factors
T-temporal factors
S-severity
medications, treatments

PMH
general health, surgeries, hospitalizations, illnesses, immunizations, medications, allergies, blood transfusions, emotional status/psychiatric history

PERSONAL HISTORY
cultural background, marital status, occupation, economic resources, environment

HEALTH HABITS
tobacco; alcohol; illicit drugs; life-style, diet, exercise; exposure to toxins

HEALTH MAINTENANCE
last PE; diagnostic tests-date, result, follow-up; self-exams-breast, genital, testicular; last Pap smear, mammogram

FAMILY HISTORY
(parents, siblings, children) cancer, DM, hypertension, heart disease, stroke

GENERAL
fever, chills, malaise, fatigue/energy, night sweats; desired weight

DIET
appetite, restrictions, vitamins, supplements

SKIN, HAIR, NAILS
rash, eruptions, itching, pigment changes

HEAD & NECK
headaches, dizziness, head injuries, loss of consciousness

EYES
blurring, double vision, visual changes, glasses, trauma, eye diseases

EARS
hearing loss, pain, discharge, vertigo, tinnitus

NOSE
congestion, nose bleeds, postnasal drip

THROAT & MOUTH
hoarseness, sore throat, bleeding gums, ulcers, tooth problems

GASTROINTESTINAL
indigestion, heartburn, vomiting, bowel regularity/changes

LYMPH
tenderness, enlargement

ENDOCRINE
heat/cold intolerance, weight change, polydipsia, polyuria, hair changes; increased hat, glove or shoe size

FEMALE
LMP, age @ menarche; gravity, parity; menses-onset, regularity, duration, symptoms, sexual life (# partners, satisfaction), contraception, menopause (age, symptoms)

MALE
puberty onset, erections, testicular pain, libido, infertility

BREASTS
pain, tenderness, lumps, discharge

CHEST & LUNGS
cough, sputum, shortness of breath, dyspnea on exertion, night sweats; exposure to TB

CARDIOVASCULAR
chest pain, palpations, number of pillows, edema, claudication, exercise tolerance

HEMATOLOGY
anemia, easy bruising

GENITOURINARY
dysuria, flank pain, urgency, frequency, nocturia, hematuria, dribbling

MUSCULOSKELETAL
joint pain, heat swelling

NEUROLOGIC
fainting, weakness, loss of coordination

MENTAL STATUS
concentration, sleeping, eating, socialization, mood changes, suicidal thoughts

PHYSICAL EXAMINATION-OBJECTIVE DATA

VS
TPR, BP, Ht, Wt

GENERAL APPEARANCE
age, race, gender, posture and gait

MENTAL STATUS
consciousness, cognitive ability, memory, emotional stability, thought content, speech quality

SKIN
color, integrity, hygiene, turgor, hydration, edema, lesions; hair distribution, texture; nail texture, nail base angle

HEAD
scalp; temporal arteries; deformities

NECK
trachea (position, tug) range of motion (ROM); carotid bruit; jugular venous distention (JVD); thyroid; lymph-head & neck

EYES
pupils (PERRLA) eyelids, conjunctivae, sclerae, EOMs (CN III, IV, VI), light reflex, visual fields, funduscopy (CN II); acuity (CN II), nystagmus

EARS
deformities, lesions, discharge, otoscopy (canal, TM), hearing (Rinne, Weber; CN VIII)

NOSE
mucosa, septum, turbinates, discharge, sinus area swelling or tenderness

MOUTH & THROAT
lips/teeth/gums, tongue (CN XII), mucosa, palates, tonsils, exudate, uvula, gag reflex (CN IX, X)

CHEST/LUNGS
shape, movement, respirations (rate, rhythm); expansion, accessory muscles, tactile fremitus, crepitus, percussion tone, excursion, auscultation (clear, wheeze, crackles, rhonchi, rubs)

BREASTS
contour, symmetry, nipples, areolae, discharge, lumps/masses; lymph-axillary, supraclavicular & infraclavicular

HEART
PMI, lifts, thrills, rate, rhythm, S1, S2, splitting, gallops, rubs, murmurs, snaps

BLOOD VESSELS
cyanosis, clubbing, edema; peripheral pulses, skin, nails

ABDOMEN
contour, symmetry, skin, bowel sounds, bruits, hum, liver span, liver border, tenderness, masses, spleen, kidneys, aortic pulsation; reflexes, percussion tone; costovertebral angle (CVA) tenderness; femoral pulses; lymph-inguinal

MALE GENITALIA
pubic hair, glans, penis, testis, scrotum, epididymis, urethral discharge, hernias

FEMALE GENITALIA
external lesions or discharge, Bartholin and Skene glands, urethra, vaginal walls, cervix (position, lesions, cervical motion tenderness), uterus, adnexae

RECTUM/PROSTATE
sacrococcygeal & perianal areas, anus, sphincter tone, rectal walls, masses, fecal occult blood test (FOBT), Male-prostate Female-rectovaginal septum, uterus

MUSCULOSKELETAL
posture, alignment, symmetry, joint heat/swelling/color; muscle tone; ROM; strength

NEUROLOGIC
CN II-XII, rapid alternating movements, finger to nose; sensation; vibration; stereognosis; motor system, gait Romberg; deep tendon reflexes (DTRs); superficial reflexes

Cranial Nerves
I-smell
II-visual acuity; visual fields, funduscopy
III, IV, VI-eyelid opening EOMs: IV up and out; VI lateral; III all others
V-corneal reflex, facial sensation (3 areas); jaw opening, bite strength
VII-eyebrow raise, eyelid close, smile, taste
VIII-Rinne, Weber
IX, X-gag reflex, palate elevation, phonation
XI-lateral head rotation, neck flexion, shoulder shrug
XII-tongue protrusion; lateral deviation strength

General Multi-system Exam - 1997

CONTENT and DOCUMENTATION REQUIREMENTS	Level of Exam	Perform and Document
	Problem Focused	One to five elements identified by a bullet.
	Expanded Problem Focused	At least six elements identified by a bullet.
	Detailed	At least two elements identified by a bullet from each of six areas/systems OR at least twelve elements identified by a bullet in two or more areas/systems.
	Comprehensive	Perform all elements identified by a bullet and document at least two elements identified by a bullet from each of nine areas/systems.

SYSTEM / BODY AREA	ELEMENTS OF EXAMINATION
Constitutional	• Measurement of any three of the following seven vital signs: 1) sitting or standing blood pressure, 2) supine blood pressure, 3) pulse rate and regularity, 4) respiration, 5) temperature, 6) height, 7) weight (may be measured and recorded by ancillary staff) • General appearance of patient e.g. development, nutrition, body habitus, deformities, attention to grooming
Eyes	• Inspection of conjunctivae and lids • Examination of pupils and irises e.g. reaction to light and accommodation, size and symmetry • Ophthalmoscopic examination of optic discs e.g. size, C/D ratio, appearance and posterior segments e.g. vessel changes, exudates, hemorrhages
Ears, nose, mouth & throat	• External inspection of ears and nose e.g. overall appearance, scars, lesions, masses • Otoscopic examination of external auditory canals and tympanic membranes • Assessment of hearing e.g. whispered voice, finger rub, tuning fork • Inspection of nasal mucosa, septum and turbinates • Inspection of lips, teeth and gums • Examination of oropharynx: oral mucosa, salivary glands, hard and soft palates, tongue, tonsils and posterior pharynx
Neck	• Examination of neck e.g. masses, overall appearance, symmetry, tracheal position, crepitus • Examination of thyroid e.g. enlargement, tenderness, mass
Respiratory	• Assessment of respiratory effort e.g. intercostal retractions, use of accessory muscles, diaphragmatic movement • Percussion of chest e.g. dullness, flatness, hyperresonance • Palpation of chest e.g. tactile fremitus • Auscultation of lungs e.g. breath sounds, adventitious sounds, rubs
Cardiovascular	• Palpation of heart e.g. location, size, thrills • Auscultation of heart with notation of abnormal sounds and murmurs Examination of: • Carotid arteries e.g. pulse amplitude, bruits, • Abdominal aorta e.g. size, bruits • Femoral arteries e.g. pulse amplitude, bruits • Pedal pulses e.g. pulse amplitude • Extremities for edema and/or varicosities
Chest (breasts)	• Inspection of breasts e.g. symmetry, nipple discharge • Palpation of breasts and axillae e.g. masses or lumps, tenderness
Gastrointestinal (abdomen)	• Examination of abdomen with notation of presence of masses or tenderness • Examination of liver and spleen • Examination for presence or absence of hernia • Examination of anus, perineum and rectum, including sphincter tone, presence of hemorrhoids, rectal masses • Obtain stool sample for occult blood test when indicated

SYSTEM / BODY AREA	ELEMENTS OF EXAMINATION
Genitourinary (male)	• Examination of the scrotal contents e.g. hydrocele, spermatocele, tenderness of cord, testicular mass • Examination of the penis • Digital rectal examination of prostate gland e.g. size, symmetry, nodularity, tenderness
Genitourinary (female)	Pelvic examination (with or without specimen collection for smears and cultures) including: • Examination of external genitalia e.g. general appearance, hair distribution, lesions and vagina e.g. general appearance, estrogen effect, discharge, lesions, pelvic support, cystocele, rectocele • Examination of the urethra e.g. masses, tenderness, scarring • Examination of the bladder e.g. fullness, masses, tenderness • Cervix e.g. general appearance, lesions, discharge • Uterus e.g. size, contour, position, mobility, tenderness, consistency, descent or support • Adnexa/parametria e.g. masses, tenderness, organomegaly, nodularity
Lymphatic	Palpation of lymph nodes in two or more areas. • Neck • Axillae • Groin • Other
Musculoskeletal	• Examination of gait and station • Inspection and/or palpations of digits and nails e.g. clubbing, cyanosis, inflammatory conditions, petechiae, ischemia, infections, nodes Examination of joints, bones and muscles of one or more of the following six areas: 1) head and neck, 2) spine, ribs and pelvis, 3) right upper extremity, 4) left upper extremity, 5) right lower extremity, 6) left lower extremity. The examination of a given area includes: • Inspection and/or palpation with notation of presence of any misalignment, asymmetry, crepitation, defects, tenderness, masses, effusions • Assessment of range of motion with notation of any pain, crepitation or contracture • Assessment of stability with notation of any dislocation (luxation), subluxation or laxity • Assessment of muscle strength and tone e.g. flaccid, cog wheel, spastic with notation of any atrophy or abnormal movements
Skin	• Inspection of skin and subcutaneous tissue e.g. rashes, lesions, ulcers • Palpation of skin and subcutaneous tissue e.g. induration, subcutaneous nodules, tightening
Neurologic	• Test cranial nerves with notation of any deficits • Examination of deep tendon reflexes with notation of pathological reflexes e.g. Babinski • Examination of sensation e.g. by touch, pin, vibration, proprioception
Psychiatric	• Description of patient's judgment and insight Brief assessment of mental status including: • Orientation to time, place and person • Recent and remote memory • Mood and affect e.g. depression, anxiety, agitation

Appendix M: HCFA-1500 Form

HEALTH INSURANCE CLAIM FORM

PLEASE DO NOT STAPLE IN THIS AREA

PLEASE PRINT OR TYPE

Appendix N: Marketing Resume

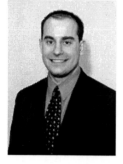

Dr. Kevin Letz
Nurse Practitioner

Board Certified: Family Nurse Practitioner (*AANP*), Pediatric Nurse Practitioner (*ANCC*), Adult Nurse Practitioner (*ANCC*), Certified Emergency Nurse (*BCEN*)

Member: American Headache Society, American Academy of Allergy, Asthma, & Immunology, American College of Allergy, Asthma, & Immunology, American Academy of Nurse Practitioners, American College of Nurse Practitioners, Coalition of Advanced Practice Nurses of Indiana

"Nurse practitioners provide quality patient care"

Nurse practitioners serve a unique role of managing both medical and nursing problems. Their practice emphasizes health promotion, illness/disease prevention, and the diagnosis and management of acute and chronic disease. Nurse practitioners conduct physical examinations, perform and interpret diagnostic testing, and prescribe medications and other treatments. Nurse practitioners are nurses with advanced graduate training allowing them to serve as primary care providers for individuals in a variety of settings.

Appendix O: Physician Consulting Agreement

THIS AGREEMENT effective _____, is between
_____NP (nurse practitioner) and
_____MD (physician).

WHEREAS, the nurse practitioner is required by law to collaborate with a licensed physician and the physician is willing to provide such collaboration.

WHEREAS, the nurse practitioner has determined that in the interest of the nurse practitioner's business, it is desirable to employ the physician for his/her professional abilities and skills.

NOW THEREFORE, for and in consideration of the mutual covenants and agreements herein set out, the parties mutually agree as follow:

TERM. The term of this Agreement shall be from
_____ to _____.

TERMINATION. The Agreement shall be terminated upon the restriction or disqualification of either party's ability to practice in the state of _____.

The Agreement shall also be determined with 90 day notification of either party.

DUTIES. The nurse practitioner shall pay the physician a sum of $_____ per contract year, with payments made on a quarterly basis.

The physician shall sign the collaboration agreement with the nurse practitioner.

The physician shall review and cosign _____% of records provided by nurse practitioner

SURVIVAL OF COVENANTS. This Agreement shall be binding upon any successors or heirs or personal representatives of the parties hereto. The covenants shall survive any termination or rescission of the Agreement unless the nurse practitioner executes a written agreement specifically releasing physician from such covenants.

CONSTRUCTION. Throughout this Agreement, the use of the singular number shall be construed to include the plural, then singular, and the use of any gender shall include all genders, whenever required by the context.

IN WITNESS WHEREOF, the Nurse Practitioner and Physician have entered into this Agreement on the day and year first above written.

Executed this ____day of _____, _____.

Physician:_____

Business address:

Nurse Practitioner:_____

Home address:

Witness:_____

Appendix P: State Boards of Nursing

Alabama   334-242-4060
770 Washington Avenue
RSA Plaza, Suite 250
Montgomery, AL 36130-3900

Alaska   907-269-8161
Department of Community and Economic Development
Division of Occupational Licensing
3601 C Street, Suite 722
Anchorage, AK 99503

Arizona   602-331-8111
1651 E. Morten Avenue, Suite 150
Phoenix, AZ 85020

Arkansas   501-686-2700
University Tower Building
1123 S. University, Suite 800
Little Rock, AR 72204-1619

California   916-322-3350
400 R Street, Suite 4030
PO Box 944210
Sacramento, CA 95814

Colorado   303-894-2430
1560 Broadway, Suite 880
Denver, CO 80202

Connecticut   860-509-7624
410 Capitol Avenue, MS# 13PHO
PO Box 340308
Hartford, CT 06134-0328

Delaware   302-739-4522
861 Silver Lake Road
Cannon Building, Suite 203
Dover, DE 19904

District of Columbia   202-442-4778
Department of Health
825 N. Capitol Street, NE 2nd Floor
Room 2224
Washington, DC 20002

Florida   904-858-6940
4080 Woodcock Drive, Suite 202
Jacksonville, FL 32207

Georgia   478-207-1640
237 Coliseum Drive
Macon, GA 31217-3858

Hawaii   808-586-3000
Professional & Vocational Licensing Division
PO Box 3469
Honolulu, HI 96801

Idaho   208-334-3110
280 N. 8th Street, Suite 210
PO Box 83720
Boise, ID 83720

Illinois   312-814-2715
James R. Thompson Center
100 West Randolph Center, Suite 9-300
Chicago, IL 60601

Indiana   317-232-2960
Health Professions Bureau
402 West Washington Street, Room W041
Indianapolis, IN 46204

Iowa   515-281-3255
River Point Business Park
400 S.W. 8th Street, Suite B
Des Moines, IA 50309-4685

Kansas   785-296-4929
Landon State Office Bldg.
900 SW Jackson, Suite 551 South

Business Essentials for Nurse Practitioners

213

Topeka, KS 66612-1230

Kentucky   502-329-7000
312 Whittington Pkwy., Suite 300
Louisville, KY 40222

Louisiana   504-838-5332
3510 N. Causeway Blvd., Suite 501
Metairie. LA 70003

Maine   207-287-1133
158 State House Station
Augusta, ME 04333

Maryland   410-585-1900
4140 Patterson Avenue
Baltimore, MD 21215

Massachusetts   617-727-9961
Commonwealth Of Massachusetts
239 Causeway Street
Boston, MA 02114

Michigan   517-373-9102
Ottawa Towers North
611 W. Ottawa, 4th Floor
Lansing, MI 48933

Minnesota   612-617-2270
2829 University Avenue, SE, Suite 500
Minneapolis, MN 55414

Mississippi   601-987-4188
1935 Lakeland Avenue, Suite B
Jackson, MS 39216-5014

Missouri   573-751-0681
3605 Missouri Blvd.
PO Box 656
Jefferson City, MO 65102-0656

Montana   406-444-2071

301 South Park
Helena, MT 59620-0513

Nebraska   402-471-4376
Department of Regulation and Licensing, Nursing Section
301 Centennial Mall South
Lincoln, NE 68509-4376

Nevada   702-486-5800
License Certification and Education
4330 S. Valley View Blvd., Suite 106
Las Vegas, NV 89103

New Hampshire 603-271-2323
PO Box 3898
78 Regional Drive, Bldg. B
Concord, NH 03302

New Jersey   973-504-6586
PO Box 45010
124 Halsey Street, 6th Floor
Newark, NJ 07101

New Mexico   505-841-8340
4206 Louisiana Blvd., NE, Suite A
Albuquerque, NM 87109

New York   518-474-3817 120
Education Bldg.
89 Washington Avenue, 2nd Floor West Wing
Albany, NY 12234

North Carolina 919-782-3211
3724 National Drive, Suite 201
Raleigh, NC 27612

North Dakota   701-328-9777
919 South 7th Street, Suite 504
Bismark, ND 58504

Ohio   614-466-3947
17 South High Street, Suite 400

Columbus, OH 43215-3413

Oklahoma   405-962-1800
2915 N. Classen Blvd., Suite 524
Oklahoma City, OK 73106

Oregon   503-731-4745
800 NE Oregon Street, Box 25, Suite 465
Portland, OR 97232

Pennsylvania   717-783-7142
124 Pine Street
Harrisburg, PA 17101

Rhode Island   401-222-5700
Registration and Nursing Education
105 Cannon Building
Three Capitol Hill
Providence, RI 02908

South Carolina   803-896-4550
110 Centerview Drive, Suite 202
Columbia, SC 29210

South Dakota   605-362-2760
4300 South Louise Ave., Suite C-1
Sioux Falls, SD 57106-3124

Tennessee   615-532-5166
426 Fifth Avenue North, 1st Floor-Cordell Hull Bldg.
Nashville, TN 37247

Texas   512-305-7400
333 Guadalupe, Suite 3-460
Austin, TX 78701

Utah   801-530-6628
Heber M. Wells Bldg., 4th Floor
160 East 300 South
Salt Lake City, UT 84111

Vermont   802-828-2396

109 State Street
Montpelier, VT 05609-1106

Virginia   804-662-9909
6606 W. Broad Street, 4th Floor
Richmond, VA 23230

Washington   360-236-4740
Department of Health
1300 Quince Street SE
Olympia, WA 98504-7864

West Virginia   304-558-3596
Board of Examiners for Registered Professional Nurses
101 Dee Drive
Charleston, WV 25311

Wisconsin   608-266-0145
1400 E. Washington Avenue
PO Box 8935
Madison, WI 53708

Wyoming   307-777-7601
2020 Carey Avenue, Suite 110
Cheyenne, WY 82002

Business Essentials for Nurse Practitioners
217

Quick Order Form

Telephone Orders: 1-260-710-0242. Have your credit card ready.

Web Orders: www.previcare.org

Postal Orders: PreviCare, Inc., 2602 Barry Knoll Way, Suite 300, Fort Wayne, IN. 46845

Please send me ___ copies of "Business Essentials for Nurse Practitioners" @ $59.99 + 4.99 S/H=$64.98

Sales tax: Please add 6% for products shipped to Indiana addresses.

Name:_____

Address:_____

City:_____ **State:**_____ **Zip:**_____

Telephone: _____

Email: _____

Please send FREE information on:

____ **Business Seminars** ____**Consulting**

Payment: ____**Check**

____**Credit Card**

____**Visa** ____**Discover** ____**Master Card**

Card Number: _____

Name on Card: _____

Expiration Date: _____

Signature: _____